Cancer Screening in Inflammatory Bowel Disease

Joseph D. Feuerstein • Adam S. Cheifetz
Editors

Cancer Screening in Inflammatory Bowel Disease

A Guide to Risk Management and Techniques

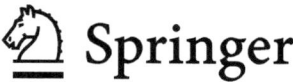 Springer

Editors
Joseph D. Feuerstein
Center for Inflammatory Bowel Disease
Beth Israel Deaconess Medical Center
Boston, MA
USA

Adam S. Cheifetz
Center for Inflammatory Bowel Disease
Beth Israel Deaconess Medical Center
Boston, MA
USA

ISBN 978-3-030-15300-7   ISBN 978-3-030-15301-4   (eBook)
https://doi.org/10.1007/978-3-030-15301-4

This Springer imprint is published by the registered company Springer Nature Switzerland AG
The registered company address is: Gewerbestrasse 11, 6330 Cham, Switzerland

Preface

Over the last two decades, the treatment of inflammatory bowel disease has evolved greatly. While historically inflammatory bowel disease (IBD) was managed with corticosteroids, 5-aminosalycilates, and thiopurines, more effective drugs including antitumor necrosis factor, anti-integrins, anti-interleukins, and Janus kinase inhibitors are now being utilized. Clinicians are now able to achieve more sustained and prolonged disease remission. Additionally, patients are living longer, and the elderly are the fastest growing segment of the population. Unfortunately, the elderly are also at the greatest risk of developing cancer, whether or not it is related to treatment of IBD. As such, clinicians need to be ever more concerned about cancer risks of IBD and the cancer risks secondary to the medications used to treat IBD and the treatment of IBD in patients with a history of cancer.

We are excited that this book, *Cancer Screening in Inflammatory Bowel Disease*, provides the readers with expert reviews on critical topics pertaining to the cancer risk associated with IBD as well as the medications used to treat the disease. This book will improve clinicians' understanding of the actual cancer risks and enable clinicians to optimize their cancer screening and surveillance of their patients with IBD.

The authors were carefully selected for their expertise in inflammatory bowel disease and their ability to succinctly summarize and explain these important concepts related to the cancer risks in IBD. Drs. Nguyen and Velayos provide an expert review of the epidemiology, risk factors, and screening for colon cancer in IBD. Drs. Kane, Lawlor, Shen, and Moss review the literature on specific cancers including lymphoma, rectal cancer, cancer following pouch formation, small bowel cancers, cholangiocarcinoma, urinary tract cancer, anal cancer, and female-specific cancer. Drs. Lichtenstein and Singh focus their chapters on cancer risks and screening with current and emerging drug therapies as well as chemoprotective approaches to reduce the risk of cancer in IBD. The final chapters authored by Drs. Kahn, Katz, and Hudesman expertly summarize the cancer risks in special situations: pediatrics, geriatrics, and the use of medications following the diagnosis of a malignancy.

We believe this book will provide the reader with a thorough review of the cancer risks associated with IBD and the medications used to treat IBD and inform the reader on how to optimize cancer screening and the care of inflammatory bowel disease.

Boston, MA, USA   Joseph D. Feuerstein
                                                                                                          Adam S. Cheifetz

Contents

Contributors

Jamie Abbott Department of Dermatology, Boston Medical Center, Boston University School of Medicine, Boston, MA, USA

Jordan Axelrad NYU School of Medicine, New York, NY, USA

Kendall Beck Division of Gastroenterology and Hepatology and Center for Crohn's and Colitis, University of California, San Francisco, San Francisco, CA, USA

Fernanda Dal Bello Division of Gastroenterology, Center for Inflammatory Bowel Disease, Beth Israel Deaconess Medical Center, Boston, MA, USA

Chip Alex Bowman Columbia University Vagelos College of Physicians and Surgeons, New York, NY, USA

Shannon Chang NYU School of Medicine, New York, NY, USA

Kara De Felice Louisiana State University Health Science Center, New Orleans, LA, USA

Francis A. Farraye Section of Gastroenterology, Boston Medical Center, Boston University School of Medicine, Boston, MA, USA

Reid L. Hopkins Section of Gastroenterology, Boston Medical Center, Boston University School of Medicine, Boston, MA, USA

David Hudesman NYU School of Medicine, New York, NY, USA

Inflammatory Bowel Disease Center, NYU Langone Health, New York, NY, USA

Stacy A. Kahn Inflammatory Bowel Disease Center, Boston Children's Hospital, Boston, MA, USA

Harvard Medical School, Boston, MA, USA

Sunanda Kane Mayo Clinic, Rochester, MN, USA

Seymour Katz New York University Langone Health, New York, NY, USA

Freeha Khan Center for Inflammatory Bowel Disease, Digestive Disease and Surgery Institute-A31, Cleveland Clinic, Cleveland, OH, USA

Matthew Kowalik Division of Gastroenterology, Hepatology and Nutrition, Boston Children's Hospital, Boston, MA, USA

Garrett Lawlor Columbia University Medical Center/NY-Presbyterian Hospital, New York, NY, USA

Helen Lee Division of Gastroenterology, Department of Medicine, Hospital of the University of Pennsylvania, Philadelphia, PA, USA

University of Pennsylvania School of Medicine, Philadelphia, PA, USA

Gary R. Lichtenstein Division of Gastroenterology, Department of Medicine, Hospital of the University of Pennsylvania, Philadelphia, PA, USA

University of Pennsylvania School of Medicine, Philadelphia, PA, USA

Center for Inflammatory Bowel Diseases, The Raymond and Ruth Perelman School of Medicine of the University of Pennsylvania, Philadelphia, PA, USA

Gastroenterology Division, Department of Internal Medicine, Perelman Center for Advanced Medicine, Philadelphia, PA, USA

Elissa Lin New York University Langone Health, New York, NY, USA

Alan C. Moss Division of Gastroenterology, Center for Inflammatory Bowel Disease, Beth Israel Deaconess Medical Center, Boston, MA, USA

Sanjay K. Murthy Department of Medicine, Division of Gastroenterology, University of Ottawa, Ottawa, ON, Canada

The Ottawa Hospital IBD Centre, Ottawa, ON, Canada

Ottawa Hospital Research Institute, Ottawa, ON, Canada

School of Epidemiology and Public Health, University of Ottawa, Ottawa, ON, Canada

Geoffrey C. Nguyen Department of Medicine, Division of Gastroenterology, University of Toronto, Toronto, ON, Canada

Mount Sinai Hospital IBD Centre, Toronto, ON, Canada

Lunenfeld-Tanenbaum Research Institute, Toronto, ON, Canada

IC/ES, Toronto, ON, Canada

Debjani Sahni Department of Dermatology, Boston Medical Center, Boston University School of Medicine, Boston, MA, USA

Yecheskel Schneider Division of Gastroenterology, Department of Medicine, Hospital of the University of Pennsylvania, Philadelphia, PA, USA

University of Pennsylvania School of Medicine, Philadelphia, PA, USA

Bo Shen Center for Inflammatory Bowel Disease, Digestive Disease and Surgery Institute-A31, Cleveland Clinic, Cleveland, OH, USA

Siddharth Singh Division of Gastroenterology, University of California San Diego, La Jolla, CA, USA

Division of Biomedical Informatics, Department of Medicine, University of California San Diego, La Jolla, CA, USA

Fernando Velayos Division of Gastroenterology and Hepatology, San Francisco Kaiser Permanente, San Francisco, CA, USA

Regional Program for Inflammatory Bowel Disease, Kaiser Permanente Northern California, Oakland, CA, USA

Chapter 1
Epidemiology and Risk Factors for Colorectal Cancer in Inflammatory Bowel Diseases

Sanjay K. Murthy and Geoffrey C. Nguyen

Introduction

Colorectal cancer (CRC) is among the most worrisome complications of colonic inflammatory bowel diseases (cIBD), accounting for up to 15% of IBD-related deaths [1]. The suspected trigger for CRC development in cIBD is chronic or recurrent mucosal inflammation, which leads to progressive DNA damage and abnormal epithelial proliferation [2]. There are differences in the timing and frequency of genetic aberrations in the dysplasia-carcinoma sequence between sporadic and IBD-associated CRC [3, 4]. Furthermore, the molecular and genetic alterations may occur more rapidly in IBD-associated CRC [3].

IBD-associated CRC has shown a propensity toward flatter and irregular growth patterns as compared to sporadic CRC, which may increase the difficulty with detecting these lesions during standard colonoscopy [5, 6]. It has even been sug-

S. K. Murthy (✉)
Department of Medicine, Division of Gastroenterology, University of Ottawa,
Ottawa, ON, Canada

The Ottawa Hospital IBD Centre, Ottawa, ON, Canada

Ottawa Hospital Research Institute, Ottawa, ON, Canada

School of Epidemiology and Public Health, University of Ottawa, Ottawa, ON, Canada
e-mail: smurthy@toh.ca

G. C. Nguyen
Department of Medicine, Division of Gastroenterology, University of Toronto,
Toronto, ON, Canada

Mount Sinai Hospital IBD Centre, Toronto, ON, Canada

Lunenfeld-Tanenbaum Research Institute, Toronto, ON, Canada

IC/ES, Toronto, ON, Canada
e-mail: geoff.nguyen@utoronto.ca

© Springer Nature Switzerland AG 2019
J. D. Feuerstein, A. S. Cheifetz (eds.), *Cancer Screening in Inflammatory Bowel Disease*, https://doi.org/10.1007/978-3-030-15301-4_1

gested that dysplastic foci in IBD patients may originate at the base of colonic crypts, which could theoretically undergo malignant transformation and progress submucosally without ever surfacing to the visible mucosa [7–9]. Further to this, molecular studies have reported widespread DNA mutations in areas of chronic colitis (termed "field carcinogenesis"), theoretically putting patients at risk of multifocal tumor development [10–12].

These observations have led to a long-held belief that IBD-associated CRC may be less detectable and less preventable than sporadic CRC, a notion supported by early observations of high rates of synchronous and metachronous CRC in persons with cIBD who had neoplastic lesions detected during colonoscopy [13–16]. Current guidelines advocate for frequent colonoscopic surveillance beginning at 8–10 years following IBD diagnosis, regardless of age [17–21]. As such, there is great interest in the epidemiology of CRC in IBD patients, particularly with respect to factors that influence CRC risk and prognosis, to help define the risk faced by patients and to better risk stratify patients for colonoscopic surveillance as well as potentially decrease future CRC risk through risk factor modification.

CRC Risk in IBD Patients

Numerous population-based and referral center studies have attempted to quantify the relative risk of CRC among IBD patients relative to members of the general population. As outlined in a recent review, this has been a challenging task due to the difficulty in quantifying multiple factors that influence CRC risk, such as time of disease onset (based on initial symptoms), burden of disease activity over time, macroscopic and microscopic colitis extent, presence and severity of comorbid conditions (such as primary sclerosing cholangitis), duration and types of medical treatments, and frequency of cancer surveillance [22]. This has led to significant heterogeneity in risk estimates across studies [22]. Population-based studies have had the advantage of sampling large heterogeneous cohorts to obtain more precise and generalizable risk estimates but have suffered from the lack of comprehensive data on risk factors to define risk in distinct subgroups of IBD patients. Referral center studies, by contrast, have typically had more comprehensive risk factor data, but have suffered from poorer generalizability and inadequate sample sizes, leading to less precise estimates of CRC risk. Other factors impacting the reliability of reported estimates of CRC risk include the low incidence of CRC in this population and lead-time bias relating to closer surveillance of IBD patients relative to persons in the general population. To date, there have been few large, well-designed studies that accurately and precisely describe the absolute and relative risk of CRC among defined subgroups of IBD patients. Furthermore, given the long lag time from IBD onset to CRC occurrence, reported risk estimates from studies typically reflect the effects of historical treatments and surveillance strategies among older cohort, which may be less indicative of the risk faced by IBD patients in the present day [22].

Relative Risk and Incidence of CRC in IBD Patients

Meta-analyses of population-based and referral center studies have defined the relative risk of CRC in IBD patients as compared with the general population [22]. Across meta-analyses of population-based studies, the pooled risk ratio for CRC is roughly 1.5- to 2-fold higher for both Crohn's disease (CD) and ulcerative colitis (UC) patients relative to matched non-IBD patients [23–27]. Meta-analyses of referral center studies have generally reported CRC risk ratios between fourfold and sixfold for IBD patients relative to non-IBD patients [23, 26–28], likely owing to greater inclusion of patients with severe and/or extensive and/or medically refractory colonic disease. A recent meta-analysis of nine population-based studies (eight reporting outcomes in UC patients [29–36] and three reporting outcomes in CD patients [30, 34, 37]) reported a pooled age- and sex-standardized incidence ratio (SIR) for CRC of 1.7 (95% CI 1.2–2.2, I^2 64%) for persons with IBD relative to members of the background population, which was the same for persons with CD and UC [27]. A contemporaneous meta-analysis of eight population-based studies [30–32, 34–36, 38, 39] in UC patients reported a risk ratio for CRC of 2.4 (95% CI 2.1–2.7, I^2 51%) relative to the background population [25].

With respect to CRC incidence, a meta-analysis of four population-based studies [30, 36, 40, 41] reported a pooled CRC incidence of 0.8% by 10 years, 2.2% by 20 years, and 4.5% for persons with more than 20 years of disease [27]. More recent population-based studies have reported an annual CRC incidence among IBD patients ranging between 0.04% and 0.1% [34, 42, 43]. By contrast, the cumulative incidence of CRC in a prospective surveillance cohort of patients with extensive UC from St. Mark's Hospital was reported to be 2.5% at 20 years, 7.6% at 30 years, and 10.8% at 40 years of disease [44].

Temporal Trends in CRC Risk

Several European and North American population-based studies have evaluated whether temporal trends in CRC risk among IBD patients have changed in parallel with improvements in IBD treatment and neoplasia surveillance strategies. While European studies have reported a declining CRC risk, North American studies have observed a stable CRC risk relative to non-IBD patients.

A population-based study from Sweden, in which 7607 persons diagnosed with IBD between 1954 and 1989 (whose diagnosis was confirmed through hospitalization or histopathology data) were linked to national hospital and cancer and death registries and followed for up to 40 years, reported a decline in relative CRC risk from fivefold during the 1960s to roughly twofold during the 2000–2004 period (*P* trend 0.006), comparing IBD patients to members of the background Swedish population and adjusting for age-, sex-, and calendar period-specific person-years of observation [34]. However, the decline was much less pronounced in more recent decades, with risk ratios relative to the background population of 2.4 (95% CI 1.8–3.1) in 1980–1989, 2.1 (95% CI 1.6–2.7) in 1990–1999, and 1.8 (95% 1.3–2.5) in 2000–2004. Comparatively, the relative risk of CRC did not decline significantly over time within the IBD cohort, adjusting for type and extent of IBD, sex, age, and time since IBD diagnosis: 1.7 (95% CI 0.6–4.4) for 1960–1969; 1.3 (95% CI 0.7–2.6) for 1970–1979; 1.2 (95% CI 0.7–2.2) for 1980–1989; and 1.1 (95% CI 0.7–1.8) for 1990–1999 (*P* trend 0.89 compared to the 2000–2004 period). These contradictory findings may partly relate to statistical power issues but could also relate to a more rapid rate of decline in CRC incidence in IBD vs. non-IBD persons in the Swedish population, even if the rate of decline within the IBD cohort itself was modest. This study further reported a significant decline in CRC-related mortality over time, both within the IBD population and when comparing IBD patients to the general population.

A Danish population-based study of 47,374 IBD patients and 7,945,116 individuals from the general population, followed for up to 30 years, reported declining age-adjusted CRC risk among UC patients relative to the general population over time (1979–1988, risk ratio 1.34, 95% CI 1.13–1.58; 1999–2008, risk ratio 0.57, 95% CI 0.41–0.80), whereas the CRC risk among CD patients relative to the general population remained stable over the same period [43]. These trends were preserved even when patients in each period were followed for a similar length of time. The overall CRC risk was not increased among persons with UC (risk ratio 1.07, 95% confidence interval [CI] 0.95–1.21) or CD (risk ratio 0.85, 95% CI 0.67–1.07) relative to the background population over the 30-year assessment period, adjusting for age, sex, and calendar year. Notably, risk estimates for CRC among IBD patients in this study may be lower than unselected IBD cohorts from other jurisdictions for several reasons. First, this study only evaluated patients who were diagnosed with IBD during the study period, and thus patients had relatively short disease duration. Additionally, colectomy rates in patients with cIBD in Denmark are three to eight times higher than in other European countries [45]. Colectomies would have been performed more often in individuals who are at higher risk for developing CRC (i.e., severe or extensive colitis, medically refractory disease, history of colorectal neoplasia, etc.). Furthermore, this study used a single IBD-related healthcare contact within administrative data to ascertain IBD patients, which has been shown to have a low specificity for IBD in other studies using health administrative data [46–48].

By contrast, a study from the Kaiser Permanente Medical Care Program, which provides comprehensive healthcare to roughly 30% of residents in Northern California, reported stable CRC rates over time in both CD and UC patients [49]. The standardized incidence of CRC among CD patients (per 100,000) was 87.9 in 1998–2001, 67.0 in 2002–2006, and 73.9 in 2007–2010 (*P* trend 0.98) and among UC patients (per 100,000) was 120.8 in 1998–2001, 62.2 in 2002–2006, and 78.6 in in 2007–2010 (*P* trend 0.40). When compared to CRC rates among 4,611,026 persons without IBD, the age- and sex-SIR of CRC was 1.6 in both CD and UC patients over the 12-year study period (95% CI 1.2–2.0 for CD, 1.3–2.0 for UC). In contrast, the CRC incidence in the general population increased by 21% over this period (*P* trend 0.0001). Notable limitations of this study are the relatively short study duration to show temporal trends in CRC risk and absence of a formal comparison of temporal trends in CRC risk in IBD vs. non-IBD patients. A notable strength of the study is that identification of IBD patients in the Kaiser Permanente database is highly accurate, with positive predictive values of 95% for any IBD, 88% for CD, and 95% for UC [50].

A study from the University of Manitoba IBD Epidemiology Database observed a nearly twofold higher risk of CRC and CRC-related mortality among IBD patients as compared to non-IBD controls matched on age, sex, and area of residence, which remained stable over the 25-year study period [51]. This study used a competing risk proportional hazards analysis and adjusted for prior lower gastrointestinal endoscopy, frequency of healthcare visits, and socioeconomic status. The adjusted hazard ratio [aHR] for CRC incidence was 2.04 (95% CI 1.29–3.22) for 1987–1993, 1.68 (95% CI 1.23–2.28) for 1994–2001, and 1.82 (95% CI 1.46–2.25) for 2002–2012. The aHR for CRC mortality was 1.48 (95% CI 0.61–3.59) for 1987–1993, 1.89 (95% CI 1.17–3.05) for 1994–2001, and 2.22 (95% CI 1.47–3.33) for 2002–2012.

Aside from the Danish study, which may represent a considerably different cohort, temporal trends in CRC risk have not declined considerably among IBD patients in different jurisdictions since the 1980s. The overall magnitude of CRC risk in IBD vs. non-IBD patients across these studies has also been comparable in recent decades. Observed differences in temporal trends between studies may simply be due to differences in study design, duration of follow-up, and patient and outcome ascertainment. Conversely, there may be real differences in IBD treatment and surveillance practice between countries that have had a greater impact on CRC risk over time in European countries. The differences in screening and surveillance practice in the general population may also have influenced these trends.

CRC-Related Mortality

Aside from a single study from Olmstead County, Minnesota, which reported no increased risk of CRC-related mortality in IBD vs. non-IBD patients [52], most studies have reported a higher mortality risk among IBD patients with CRC, with risk ratios ranging between 1.2- and 2-fold across population-based studies from North America, Europe, and Japan [34, 49, 51, 53, 54]. These findings parallel the higher CRC risk among IBD patients as compared to non-IBD patients. A study from Japan reported poorer 5-year survival with advanced CRC (Stage III) in UC patients (43.3%) as compared to non-IBD patients (57.4%) (aHR for death 2.0, 95% CI 1.2–3.3), adjusting for age, gender, and year of cancer diagnosis [55]. However, there was no significant difference in the 5-year overall survival rate between the UC-CRC (64.2%) and the sporadic CRC (68.7%) groups. A population-based study from Sweden further reported declining risk CRC-related mortality over time among IBD patients [34]. Conversely, a population-based study from Manitoba, Canada, did not observe a change in CRC-related mortality over a 25-year period [51].

CRC Risk Factors

Disease Duration

Disease duration has long been recognized as an important factor predicting CRC risk in persons with cIBD. National societies advocate commencing CRC screening in these patients at 8–10 years following disease diagnosis, based on epidemiologic trends for CRC risk [17–21]. Some guidelines further recommend more frequent surveillance as the disease duration progresses [18, 19, 21].

A large meta-analysis of single-center and population-based studies pre-dating the twenty-first century reported a cumulative CRC incidence of roughly 8% by 20 years and 18% by 30 years of disease among UC patients [28]. A meta-analysis of four population-based studies in persons with cIBD, three from Scandinavia [36, 40, 41] and one from USA [30], reported a pooled CRC risk of 0.8% (95% CI 0.4–1.4%) by 10 years, 2.2% (95% CI 0.8–2.4%) by 20 years, and 4.5% (95% CI 0.8–7.2%) beyond 20 years [27]. Another meta-analysis of population-based studies in UC patients that included two of the cohorts in the prior meta-analysis [30, 36], four additional Scandinavian cohorts [31, 34, 35, 39], an Italian cohort [32], and a Canadian cohort [38] reported a cumulative CRC incidence across individual studies of 1.0% at 10 years 0.4–2% at 15 years, and 1.1–5.3% at 20 years of follow-up [25]. As most of these studies evaluated historical cohorts predating the introduction of biological therapy, the use of routine objective markers of inflammation, and treating to a target of mucosal healing, these rates may overestimate the effect of disease duration on CRC risk in modern-day IBD cohorts.

Population-based studies in more recent cohorts reporting long-term follow-up have reported similar trends for CRC risk with respect to duration of disease. A Dutch study of IBD patients from 78 (out of 93) general hospitals between 1990 and 2006 found that patients with greater than 20 years of disease had a risk ratio of 4.42 (95% CI 3.07–6.36) for development of CRC when compared with patients with less than 10 years of disease [42]. Disease duration was independently associated with CRC risk (risk ratio of 1.04 (95% CI 1.02–1.05) per year of IBD) after adjusting for age, sex, colonic disease extent, presence of PSC, and presence of pseudopolyposis.

A Danish population-based study of IBD patients diagnosed between 1979 and 2008 found a gradual increase in CRC risk with duration of disease in UC patients, but not in CD patients [43]. Risk of CRC in UC patients increased significantly over background risk beyond 13 years following diagnosis to reach a steady-state risk ratio of roughly 1.5. CRC risk in patients with CD did not deviate significantly from background risk even after 20 years of disease, although the authors did not specifically evaluate CD patients with colonic disease. Again, inclusion of only incident IBD cases and high colectomy rates among IBD patients in Denmark may have resulted in lower estimates of CRC risk as compared to what might be seen into unselected cohorts from other jurisdictions.

In a study of a prospective surveillance cohort of patients with extensive UC from St. Mark's Hospital that underwent annual or biannual colonoscopy with random and targeted biopsies, the cumulative incidence of CRC was 2.5% at 20 years, 7.6% at 30 years, and 10.8% at 40 years [44].

Extent of Colitis

Colonic disease extent is also recognized as an important factor predicting CRC risk among IBD patients and has been advocated as a risk-stratifying feature for neoplasia surveillance by multiple societies [17–19, 21]. A major difficulty with quantifying the impact of colitis extent on CRC risk is that it changes in a substantial proportion of persons over time [56, 57]. However, most studies have quantified disease extent at a specific point of time in the IBD disease course (i.e., at diagnosis or at study entry), thereby ignoring the specific contributions of varying extent of colitis over time. An additional challenge is to quantify colitis extent as whether microscopic extent or macroscopic colitis extent, which does not always correlate with one another.

A landmark population-based study of 3117 Swedish patients diagnosed with UC between 1922 and 1983 initially characterized the importance of colitis extent as a predictor of CRC risk, showing that patients with pancolitis at diagnosis had close to a 15-fold excess CRC risk relative to the background population (SIR 14.8, 95% CI 11.4–18.9), whereas those with left-sided colitis at diagnosis had just five-fold excess CRC risk (SIR 2.8, 95% CI 1.6–4.4) and those with isolated proctitis had no excess CRC risk (SIR 1.7, 95% CI 0.8–3.2).

A recent meta-analysis has summarized important population-based and referral center studies reporting CRC risk among persons with IBD relative to the background population, stratified by disease extent [27]. Overall, persons with extensive colitis carry a substantially higher risk of developing CRC relative to matched patients from the general population, whereas those with limited colonic involvement generally do not demonstrate a significantly higher CRC risk over background.

Disease Severity

It is widely believed that inflammation is the cornerstone of CRC development in persons with cIBD [58]. As such, it could be reasonably inferred that severity of inflammation should correlate with CRC risk, even though surprisingly little data exist to support this notion. It might also be inferred that the decreasing CRC risk observed among IBD patients in some studies could be partly due to the improved treatments having reduced the overall colitis burden among IBD patients over time. As with disease extent, the severity of inflammatory disease activity can be difficult to quantify as it varies over time and depends on whether macroscopic or microscopic inflammation is evaluated. Furthermore, total inflammatory burden may not be easily discernible based on the endoscopic or histological appearance of inflammation alone, as these do not capture submucosal involvement, particularly in persons with CD. Indeed, post-inflammatory polyposis, colonic strictures, colonic foreshortening, and need for immunosuppressive therapy may all be indirect signs of severe inflammatory burden over time.

In a study from the Mayo Clinic, in which 188 patients with UC-related CRC were matched to controls based on gender, maximal extent of colitis, duration of colitis, date of first UC clinic visit, and calendar year of UC diagnosis, the presence of post-inflammatory polyps (adjusted odds ratio [aOR], 2.5; 95% CI 1.4–4.6), use of corticosteroids (aOR, 0.4; 95% CI 0.2–0.8), and use of 5-aminosalicylic acid agents (aOR, 0.4; 95% CI 0.2–0.9) were all independently associated with CRC risk, after adjusting for age at colitis diagnosis and colitis duration [59]. Other significantly associated factors were having had one or two surveillance colonoscopies (aOR, 0.4; 95% CI 0.2–0.7), history of smoking (aOR, 0.5; 95% CI 0.2–0.9), use of aspirin (aOR, 0.3; 95% CI 0.1–0.8), and use of nonsteroidal anti-inflammatory drugs (aOR, 0.1; 95% CI 0.03–0.5). Notably, history of thiopurine use and presence of primary sclerosing cholangitis were not associated with CRC risk in this study.

A case-control study from a prospective surveillance cohort of patients with long-standing extensive UC from St. Mark's Hospital, in which 68 patients with neoplasia detected during colonoscopy (dysplasia or cancer) were matched to 136 controls without neoplasia by sex, age at onset of colitic symptoms, and duration and extent of UC, found that post-inflammatory polyps (aOR 2.29, 95% CI 1.28–4.11) and colonic strictures (aOR 4.62, 95% CI 1.03–20.8) were independently associated with an increased likelihood of neoplasia detection [44]. Conversely, a macroscopically normal-appearing colon (aOR 0.38, 95% CI 0.19–0.73) was associated with a decreased risk of neoplasia detection. Having a shortened colon, a tubular-appearing colon or a segment of severe inflammation was also associated with an increased risk of harboring neoplasia in this population, although not in multivariable analysis.

Using the same cohort and study design, the investigators further assessed the association between segmental macroscopic and microscopic colonic inflammation and CRC risk, using a 5-point scale to quantify the severity of inflammation. Both parameters were significantly associated with CRC risk, but only histological severity was independently associated with CRC risk (aOR, 4.7; $p < 0.001$) [60].

In a study from the University of Chicago, in which 59 patients with UC who developed colorectal neoplasia were matched by age, disease extent, and disease duration to 141 patients with UC who did not develop colorectal neoplasia, histological inflammatory activity was independently associated with CRC risk (aOR per unit increase in mean histological score 3.68; $p = 0.001$) based on a 6-point histological scoring system developed by the investigators [61]. Use of immune modulators (aOR 0.25, 95% CI 0.08–0.73) and mesalamine (aOR 0.37, 95% CI 0.13–1.04) was negatively associated with CRC risk, while male gender was positively associated with CRC risk (aOR 5.45, 95% CI 1.79–16.6).

In a retrospective review of 418 UC patients undergoing regular endoscopic surveillance for dysplasia at Mount Sinai Hospital, New York, of whom 65 developed colorectal neoplasia and 15 developed advanced neoplasia (high-grade dysplasia or CRC), histological inflammation, assessed using a 4-point scale and analyzed as a time-varying covariate, was a significant predictor of future development of advanced neoplasia (hazard ratio (HR), 3.8; 95% CI 1.7–8.6), adjusting for prior colonoscopy exposure (which was the only other significant variable) [62].

Age at IBD Diagnosis

Age is a well-accepted risk factor for most cancers in the general population. Increasing age has also been shown to be a risk factor for CRC among persons with cIBD [42, 63]; however, IBD-associated CRC affects patients at a younger age than sporadic CRC. A meta-analysis of 116 studies predating the year 2000 reported the mean age of CRC diagnosis in IBD patients to be 43.2 years [28]. Interestingly, a population-based study from Sweden found a higher cumulative incidence of CRC, over 25 years of observation, among persons diagnosed with ulcerative pancolitis between 0 and 14 years of age as compared to those diagnosed with this condition between 15 and 39 years of age [40]. Greater censoring of deaths due to other causes in the older age group may have factored into this finding. Notably, persons aged 40 or older at diagnosis had a substantially higher cumulative probability of CRC by 20 years (end of follow-up in this group) than either of the younger age groups.

Most studies have evaluated the relative risk of CRC for different age groups at IBD diagnosis relative to the background risk in those age groups. A meta-analysis of five population-based studies [30, 37, 39–41] showed a pooled SIR for CRC of 8.2 (95% CI 1.8–14.6, I^2 82%) among persons aged less than 30 at IBD diagnosis and 1.8 (0.9–2.7, I^2 81%) among persons aged 30 or older at diagnosis [27]. Among three referral center studies [64–66], the pooled SIRs for these age groups were 70.7 (95% CI 15.6–320.9, I^2 90%) and 5.5 (95% CI 2.0–14.9, I^2 84%), respectively [27]. Other meta-analyses have reported similar findings [25]. Higher relative risk of CRC in younger IBD persons likely relates as much to low baseline CRC risk in young persons as it does to longer duration of inflammatory disease in these persons relative to older persons.

A population-based study from Denmark similarly demonstrated that young age at UC diagnosis is associated with a higher relative risk of CRC. Among patients diagnosed with UC in childhood or adolescence (0–19 years), the SIR was 43.8 (95% CI 27.2–70.7); among those diagnosed in young adulthood (20–39 years), the SIR was 2.65 (95% CI 1.97–3.56); and among those diagnosed in older age (60 and 79), the risk was lower than the background population (SIR 0.76, 95% CI 0.62–

0.92) [43]. High colectomy rates among IBD patients in Denmark may have partly accounted for the latter finding [45].

Overall, it is conceivable that cIBD diagnosis at a very young age (i.e., teens or 20s) could confer a greater long-term susceptibility to developing CRC as compared with diagnosis in early to mid- adulthood, due to a longer period of inflammatory disease during a time when inherent CRC risk is low. However, as patients enter their middle years and older age, age-related CRC risk likely becomes a dominant factor.

Sex

A meta-analysis of four population-based studies [30, 38, 39, 67] in UC patients reported pooled estimates for SIR of CRC of 1.9 (95% CI 1.5–2.3) in women and 2.6 (95% CI 2.2–3.0) in men [25]. A contemporaneous meta-analysis [27] of studies of patients with either CD or UC reported pooled SIR of 1.9 (95% CI 0.8–3.0) in males and 1.4 (95% CI 0.8–2.1) in females across three population-based studies [30, 31, 67] and SIR of 6.7 (95% CI 0.3–13.1) in males and 6.9 (95% CI 2.7–11.7) in females across three referral center studies [64, 68, 69]. Overall, males with IBD may carry a marginally higher relative risk of CRC than females.

Family History

Sporadic CRC in relatives has been associated with roughly a twofold increased risk of CRC among persons with IBD [70, 71]. A population-based study from Sweden, in which pathologically confirmed cases of CD or UC were linked to national generation and cancer registries, reported an adjusted rate ratio (aRR) of CRC of 2.5 (95% CI 1.4–4.4) for all IBD patients, 2.0 (95% CI 1.0–4.1) for those with UC, and 3.7 (1.4–9.4) for those with CD, comparing persons with a family history of sporadic CRC to those without and adjusting for age, sex, and calendar period. Patients with a first-degree relative diagnosed with CRC before 50 years of age had a higher aRR (9.2, 95% CI 3.7–23) as compared to those with a first-degree relative diagnosed with CRC after age 50 (aRR 1.7, 95% CI 0.8–3.4). Another referral center study, in which 147 UC patients diagnosed with CRC were compared to 150 UC patients without CRC, reported an aOR of 2.33 (95% CI 1.06–5.14) for development of CRC among IBD patients that had a first-degree relative with CRC as compared to those that did not, adjusting for age, sex, and UC duration.

Primary Sclerosing Cholangitis (PSC)

The risk of colorectal cancer is higher in patients with UC and PSC compared to those with UC alone, especially for right-sided colon cancer. Data on the risk of CRC in patients with CD and PSC are scarce. A Swedish population-based cohort study in 125 patients with verified diagnoses of UC and PSC reported a cumulative incidence of CRC of 16% by 10 years [72]. A French referral cohort of 75 PSC-IBD patients compared to 150 IBD patients without PSC, matched for sex, birth date, IBD diagnosis date, and initial disease location, reported a 25-year cumulative rate of CRC of 23.4% in PSC-IBD patients as compared to 0% in controls ($p = 0.002$) [73]. PSC was the only independent risk factor for the development of colorectal cancer in this study (aOR 10.8, 95% CI 3.7–31.3).

A meta-analysis of 11 studies in UC patients found a summary odds ratio of 4.09 (95% CI 2.89–5.76) for CRC among patients with PSC as compared to those without PSC [74]. In a recent population-based study from Denmark, comprising 32,911 patients with UC and 14,463 patients with CD followed for up to 30 years, of whom 6268 had PSC, presence of PSC was a strong risk factor for CRC development in UC (risk ratio 9.13, 95% CI 4.52–18.5) but not in CD (RR, 2.90, 95% CI 0.40–20.9), adjusting for age, sex, and calendar time [43]. Among IBD patients with PSC, the median time from IBD diagnosis to CRC was 13.7 years, whereas the median time from PSC diagnosis to CRC in these patients was only 1.3 years. All cases of CRC among IBD patients with PSC were right-sided colon cancers as compared with only 38% of cases of CRC among IBD patients without PSC.

The reasons for a higher CRC risk in IBD patients with PSC are unclear but may partly relate to the fact that these patients typically have pancolitis and a long period of quiescent disease by the time of diagnosis [75]. The latter may relate to a long subclinical phase of PSC before cholestatic symptoms develop (e.g., 10–15 years) [76], coupled with the relatively quiescent course of colitis in these patients [75]. There is debate as to whether alterations in bile acid secretion and/or composition play a role in CRC development in IBD patients with PSC [77]. Interestingly, a meta-analysis of eight studies found a significant negative association between ursodeoxycholic acid (UDCA) and advanced CRN (colorectal cancer and/or high-grade dysplasia) (summary OR 0.35, 95% CI 0.17–0.73) and between low-dose UDCA (8–15 mg/kg/d) and colorectal neoplasia in patients with IBD (summary OR 0.19, 95% CI 0.08–0.49), potentially implicating a role of bile acids in CRC pathogenesis [78].

References

1. Munkholm P. Review article: the incidence and prevalence of colorectal cancer in inflammatory bowel disease. Aliment Pharmacol Ther. 2003;18(Suppl 2):1–5.
2. Murthy S, Flanigan A, Clearfield H. Colorectal cancer in inflammatory bowel disease: molecular and clinical features. Gastroenterol Clin N Am. 2002;31:551–64, x.
3. Zisman TL, Rubin DT. Colorectal cancer and dysplasia in inflammatory bowel disease. World J Gastroenterol. 2008;14:2662–9.
4. Rhodes JM, Campbell BJ. Inflammation and colorectal cancer: IBD-associated and sporadic cancer compared. Trends Mol Med. 2002;8:10–6.
5. Rutter MD. Importance of nonpolypoid (flat and depressed) colorectal neoplasms in screening for CRC in patients with IBD. Gastrointest Endosc Clin N Am. 2014;24:327–35.

6. Tytgat GN, Dhir V, Gopinath N. Endoscopic appearance of dysplasia and cancer in inflammatory bowel disease. Eur J Cancer. 1995;31A:1174–7.
7. Low D, Mino-Kenudson M, Mizoguchi E. Recent advancement in understanding colitis-associated tumorigenesis. Inflamm Bowel Dis. 2014;20:2115–23.
8. Matkowskyj KA, Chen ZE, Rao MS, Yang GY. Dysplastic lesions in inflammatory bowel disease: molecular pathogenesis to morphology. Arch Pathol Lab Med. 2013;137:338–50.
9. Rubio CA, Slezak P. The unique pathology of nonpolypoid colorectal neoplasia in IBD. Gastrointest Endosc Clin N Am. 2014;24:455–68.
10. Lofberg R, Brostrom O, Karlen P, Ost A, Tribukait B. DNA aneuploidy in ulcerative colitis: reproducibility, topographic distribution, and relation to dysplasia. Gastroenterology. 1992;102:1149–54.
11. Lyda MH, Noffsinger A, Belli J, Fischer J, Fenoglio-Preiser CM. Multifocal neoplasia involving the colon and appendix in ulcerative colitis: pathological and molecular features. Gastroenterology. 1998;115:1566–73.
12. Rubin CE, Haggitt RC, Burmer GC, et al. DNA aneuploidy in colonic biopsies predicts future development of dysplasia in ulcerative colitis. Gastroenterology. 1992;103:1611–20.
13. Bernstein CN, Shanahan F, Weinstein WM. Are we telling patients the truth about surveillance colonoscopy in ulcerative colitis? Lancet. 1994;343:71–4.
14. Connell WR, Talbot IC, Harpaz N, et al. Clinicopathological characteristics of colorectal carcinoma complicating ulcerative colitis. Gut. 1994;35:1419–23.
15. Lindberg B, Persson B, Veress B, Ingelman-Sundberg H, Granqvist S. Twenty years' colonoscopic surveillance of patients with ulcerative colitis. Detection of dysplastic and malignant transformation. Scand J Gastroenterol. 1996;31:1195–204.
16. Thomas T, Abrams KA, Robinson RJ, Mayberry JF. Meta-analysis: cancer risk of low-grade dysplasia in chronic ulcerative colitis. Aliment Pharmacol Ther. 2007;25:657–68.
17. Cairns SR, Scholefield JH, Steele RJ, et al. Guidelines for colorectal cancer screening and surveillance in moderate and high risk groups (update from 2002). Gut. 2010;59:666–89.
18. Farraye FA, Odze RD, Eaden J, et al. AGA medical position statement on the diagnosis and management of colorectal neoplasia in inflammatory bowel disease. Gastroenterology. 2010;138:738–45.
19. Itzkowitz SH, Present DH. Consensus conference: colorectal cancer screening and surveillance in inflammatory bowel disease. Inflamm Bowel Dis. 2005;11:314–21.
20. Kornbluth A, Sachar DB. Ulcerative colitis practice guidelines in adults: American College of Gastroenterology, Practice Parameters Committee. Am J Gastroenterol. 2010;105:501–23.
21. Leddin D, Hunt R, Champion M, et al. Canadian Association of Gastroenterology and the Canadian Digestive Health Foundation: guidelines on colon cancer screening. Can J Gastroenterol. 2004;18:93–9.
22. Adami HO, Bretthauer M, Emilsson L, et al. The continuing uncertainty about cancer risk in inflammatory bowel disease. Gut. 2016;65:889–93.
23. Castano-Milla C, Chaparro M, Gisbert JP. Systematic review with meta-analysis: the declining risk of colorectal cancer in ulcerative colitis. Aliment Pharmacol Ther. 2014;39:645–59.
24. Jess T, Gamborg M, Matzen P, Munkholm P, Sorensen TI. Increased risk of intestinal cancer in Crohn's disease: a meta-analysis of population-based cohort studies. Am J Gastroenterol. 2005;100:2724–9.
25. Jess T, Rungoe C, Peyrin-Biroulet L. Risk of colorectal cancer in patients with ulcerative colitis: a meta-analysis of population-based cohort studies. Clin Gastroenterol Hepatol. 2012;10:639–45.
26. Laukoetter MG, Mennigen R, Hannig CM, et al. Intestinal cancer risk in Crohn's disease: a meta-analysis. J Gastrointest Surg. 2011;15:576–83.
27. Lutgens MW, van Oijen MG, van der Heijden GJ, Vleggaar FP, Siersema PD, Oldenburg B. Declining risk of colorectal cancer in inflammatory bowel disease: an updated meta-analysis of population-based cohort studies. Inflamm Bowel Dis. 2013;19:789–99.
28. Eaden JA, Abrams KR, Mayberry JF. The risk of colorectal cancer in ulcerative colitis: a meta-analysis. Gut. 2001;48:526–35.

29. Gilat T, Fireman Z, Grossman A, et al. Colorectal cancer in patients with ulcerative colitis. A population study in central Israel. Gastroenterology. 1988;94:870–7.
30. Jess T, Loftus EV Jr, Velayos FS, et al. Risk of intestinal cancer in inflammatory bowel disease: a population-based study from Olmsted County, Minnesota. Gastroenterology. 2006;130:1039–46.
31. Jess T, Riis L, Vind I, et al. Changes in clinical characteristics, course, and prognosis of inflammatory bowel disease during the last 5 decades: a population-based study from Copenhagen, Denmark. Inflamm Bowel Dis. 2007;13:481–9.
32. Palli D, Trallori G, Bagnoli S, et al. Hodgkin's disease risk is increased in patients with ulcerative colitis. Gastroenterology. 2000;119:647–53.
33. Rutegard JN, Ahsgren LR, Janunger KG. Ulcerative colitis. Colorectal cancer risk in an unselected population. Ann Surg. 1988;208:721–4.
34. Soderlund S, Brandt L, Lapidus A, et al. Decreasing time-trends of colorectal cancer in a large cohort of patients with inflammatory bowel disease. Gastroenterology. 2009;136:1561–7.
35. Stewenius J, Adnerhill I, Anderson H, et al. Incidence of colorectal cancer and all cause mortality in non-selected patients with ulcerative colitis and indeterminate colitis in Malmo, Sweden. Int J Color Dis. 1995;10:117–22.
36. Wandall EP, Damkier P, Moller Pedersen F, Wilson B, Schaffalitzky de Muckadell OB. Survival and incidence of colorectal cancer in patients with ulcerative colitis in Funen county diagnosed between 1973 and 1993. Scand J Gastroenterol. 2000;35:312–7.
37. Jess T, Winther KV, Munkholm P, Langholz E, Binder V. Intestinal and extra-intestinal cancer in Crohn's disease: follow-up of a population-based cohort in Copenhagen County, Denmark. Aliment Pharmacol Ther. 2004;19:287–93.
38. Bernstein CN, Blanchard JF, Kliewer E, Wajda A. Cancer risk in patients with inflammatory bowel disease: a population-based study. Cancer. 2001;91:854–62.
39. Winther KV, Jess T, Langholz E, Munkholm P, Binder V. Long-term risk of cancer in ulcerative colitis: a population-based cohort study from Copenhagen County. Clin Gastroenterol Hepatol. 2004;2:1088–95.
40. Ekbom A, Helmick C, Zack M, Adami HO. Ulcerative colitis and colorectal cancer. A population-based study. N Engl J Med. 1990;323:1228–33.
41. Ekbom A, Helmick C, Zack M, Adami HO. Increased risk of large-bowel cancer in Crohn's disease with colonic involvement. Lancet. 1990;336:357–9.
42. Baars JE, Looman CW, Steyerberg EW, et al. The risk of inflammatory bowel disease-related colorectal carcinoma is limited: results from a nationwide nested case-control study. Am J Gastroenterol. 2011;106:319–28.
43. Jess T, Simonsen J, Jorgensen KT, Pedersen BV, Nielsen NM, Frisch M. Decreasing risk of colorectal cancer in patients with inflammatory bowel disease over 30 years. Gastroenterology. 2012;143:375–81.
44. Rutter MD, Saunders BP, Wilkinson KH, et al. Thirty-year analysis of a colonoscopic surveillance program for neoplasia in ulcerative colitis. Gastroenterology. 2006;130:1030–8.
45. Hoie O, Wolters FL, Riis L, et al. Low colectomy rates in ulcerative colitis in an unselected European cohort followed for 10 years. Gastroenterology. 2007;132:507–15.
46. Benchimol EI, Guttmann A, Griffiths AM, et al. Increasing incidence of paediatric inflammatory bowel disease in Ontario, Canada: evidence from health administrative data. Gut. 2009;58:1490–7.
47. Benchimol EI, Guttmann A, Mack DR, et al. Validation of international algorithms to identify adults with inflammatory bowel disease in health administrative data from Ontario, Canada. J Clin Epidemiol. 2014;67:887–96.
48. Bernstein CN, Blanchard JF, Rawsthorne P, Wajda A. Epidemiology of Crohn's disease and ulcerative colitis in a central Canadian province: a population-based study. Am J Epidemiol. 1999;149:916–24.
49. Herrinton LJ, Liu L, Levin TR, Allison JE, Lewis JD, Velayos F. Incidence and mortality of colorectal adenocarcinoma in persons with inflammatory bowel disease from 1998 to 2010. Gastroenterology. 2012;143:382–9.

50. Herrinton LJ, Liu L, Lewis JD, Griffin PM, Allison J. Incidence and prevalence of inflammatory bowel disease in a Northern California managed care organization, 1996–2002. Am J Gastroenterol. 2008;103:1998–2006.
51. Singh H, Nugent Z, Lix L, Targownik L, Samadder NJ, Bernstein CN. There is no decrease in the mortality from IBD associated colorectal cancers over 25 years: a population based analysis. Gastroenterology. 2016;150:S226–S7.
52. Delaunoit T, Limburg PJ, Goldberg RM, Lymp JF, Loftus EV Jr. Colorectal cancer prognosis among patients with inflammatory bowel disease. Clin Gastroenterol Hepatol. 2006;4:335–42.
53. Ording AG, Horvath-Puho E, Erichsen R, et al. Five-year mortality in colorectal cancer patients with ulcerative colitis or Crohn's disease: a nationwide population-based cohort study. Inflamm Bowel Dis. 2013;19:800–5.
54. Watanabe T, Ajioka Y, Mitsuyama K, et al. Comparison of targeted vs random biopsies for surveillance of ulcerative colitis-associated colorectal cancer. Gastroenterology. 2016;151:1122–30.
55. Watanabe T, Konishi T, Kishimoto J, Kotake K, Muto T, Sugihara K. Ulcerative colitis-associated colorectal cancer shows a poorer survival than sporadic colorectal cancer: a nationwide Japanese study. Inflamm Bowel Dis. 2011;17:802–8.
56. Roda G, Narula N, Pinotti R, et al. Systematic review with meta-analysis: proximal disease extension in limited ulcerative colitis. Aliment Pharmacol Ther. 2017;45:1481–92.
57. Safroneeva E, Vavricka S, Fournier N, et al. Systematic analysis of factors associated with progression and regression of ulcerative colitis in 918 patients. Aliment Pharmacol Ther. 2015;42:540–8.
58. Shanahan F. Relation between colitis and colon cancer. Lancet. 2001;357:246–7.
59. Velayos FS, Loftus EV Jr, Jess T, et al. Predictive and protective factors associated with colorectal cancer in ulcerative colitis: a case-control study. Gastroenterology. 2006;130:1941–9.
60. Rutter M, Saunders B, Wilkinson K, et al. Severity of inflammation is a risk factor for colorectal neoplasia in ulcerative colitis. Gastroenterology. 2004;126:451–9.
61. Rubin DT, Huo D, Kinnucan JA, et al. Inflammation is an independent risk factor for colonic neoplasia in patients with ulcerative colitis: a case-control study. Clin Gastroenterol Hepatol. 2013;11:1601–8.e1–4.
62. Gupta RB, Harpaz N, Itzkowitz S, et al. Histologic inflammation is a risk factor for progression to colorectal neoplasia in ulcerative colitis: a cohort study. Gastroenterology. 2007;133:1099–105; quiz 340–1.
63. Karvellas CJ, Fedorak RN, Hanson J, Wong CK. Increased risk of colorectal cancer in ulcerative colitis patients diagnosed after 40 years of age. Can J Gastroenterol. 2007;21:443–6.
64. Macdougall IP. The cancer risk in ulcerative colitis. Lancet. 1964;2:655–8.
65. Gillen CD, Walmsley RS, Prior P, Andrews HA, Allan RN. Ulcerative colitis and Crohn's disease: a comparison of the colorectal cancer risk in extensive colitis. Gut. 1994;35:1590–2.
66. Gyde SN, Prior P, Allan RN, et al. Colorectal cancer in ulcerative colitis: a cohort study of primary referrals from three centres. Gut. 1988;29:206–17.
67. Soderlund S, Granath F, Brostrom O, et al. Inflammatory bowel disease confers a lower risk of colorectal cancer to females than to males. Gastroenterology. 2010;138:1697–703.
68. Prior P, Gyde SN, Macartney JC, Thompson H, Waterhouse JA, Allan RN. Cancer morbidity in ulcerative colitis. Gut. 1982;23:490–7.
69. Gyde SN, Prior P, Macartney JC, Thompson H, Waterhouse JA, Allan RN. Malignancy in Crohn's disease. Gut. 1980;21:1024–9.
70. Askling J, Dickman PW, Karlen P, et al. Family history as a risk factor for colorectal cancer in inflammatory bowel disease. Gastroenterology. 2001;120:1356–62.
71. Nuako KW, Ahlquist DA, Mahoney DW, Schaid DJ, Siems DM, Lindor NM. Familial predisposition for colorectal cancer in chronic ulcerative colitis: a case-control study. Gastroenterology. 1998;115:1079–83.
72. Kornfeld D, Ekbom A, Ihre T. Is there an excess risk for colorectal cancer in patients with ulcerative colitis and concomitant primary sclerosing cholangitis? A population based study. Gut. 1997;41:522–5.

73. Sokol H, Cosnes J, Chazouilleres O, et al. Disease activity and cancer risk in inflammatory bowel disease associated with primary sclerosing cholangitis. World J Gastroenterol. 2008;14:3497–503.
74. Soetikno RM, Lin OS, Heidenreich PA, Young HS, Blackstone MO. Increased risk of colorectal neoplasia in patients with primary sclerosing cholangitis and ulcerative colitis: a meta-analysis. Gastrointest Endosc. 2002;56:48–54.
75. Broome U, Bergquist A. Primary sclerosing cholangitis, inflammatory bowel disease, and colon cancer. Semin Liver Dis. 2006;26:31–41.
76. Aadland E, Schrumpf E, Fausa O, et al. Primary sclerosing cholangitis: a long-term follow-up study. Scand J Gastroenterol. 1987;22:655–64.
77. Blackstone MO. An association of fecal bile acids and colon cancer in ulcerative colitis? Gastroenterology. 1988;95:575–6.
78. Singh S, Khanna S, Pardi DS, Loftus EV Jr, Talwalkar JA. Effect of ursodeoxycholic acid use on the risk of colorectal neoplasia in patients with primary sclerosing cholangitis and inflammatory bowel disease: a systematic review and meta-analysis. Inflamm Bowel Dis. 2013;19:1631–8.

Chapter 2
Screening for Colon Cancer in Inflammatory Bowel Disease

Kendall Beck and Fernando Velayos

Introduction

The development of colorectal cancer (CRC) is one of the most dreaded complications of long-standing inflammatory bowel disease (IBD) [1]. The first case report of such an occurrence was published by Crohn and Rosenberg in 1925 [2]. It described a case of rectal cancer occurring within an area of long-standing inflammation despite the patient being under the expert and close care of these physicians. Since then, the question of how to prevent colorectal cancer in patients with IBD has been a unique challenge. The literature has shown the limitations of screening for precancerous lesions as they can be promoted and obscured by inflammation and occur despite expert and close care.

How to Prevent Colorectal Cancer in IBD

The answer of how to prevent colorectal cancer in IBD (or any condition) is to apply an effective screening test that can detect the condition at a preclinical and intervenable state that impacts outcome. Prior to the advent of colonoscopy, the options for

K. Beck (✉)
Division of Gastroenterology and Hepatology and Center for Crohn's and Colitis,
University of California, San Francisco, San Francisco, CA, USA
e-mail: Kendall.Beck@ucsf.edu

F. Velayos
Division of Gastroenterology and Hepatology, San Francisco Kaiser Permanente,
San Francisco, CA, USA

Regional Program for Inflammatory Bowel Disease, Kaiser Permanente Northern California,
Oakland, CA, USA
e-mail: Fernando.Velayos@kp.org

© Springer Nature Switzerland AG 2019
J. D. Feuerstein, A. S. Cheifetz (eds.), *Cancer Screening in Inflammatory Bowel Disease*, https://doi.org/10.1007/978-3-030-15301-4_2

colorectal cancer screening in IBD were limited (physical exam, proctoscopy, and barium enema). Case reports published during this time reinforced the lack of effective screening options by highlighting the development of colorectal cancer despite regular care for IBD [2–4]. Perhaps not surprisingly, prophylactic proctocolectomy was advocated for many decades as the most effective way of preventing colorectal cancer in this high-risk population due to the absence of effective screening options and interventions.

Even after the advent of colonoscopy, how physicians view the effectiveness of colonoscopy as a screening exam has evolved over the past 50 years. Advances in optical technology (fiber optics, then standard definition, and now high definition), improvements in bowel preparation (single dose to now split-dose preparation), recognition of flat polyps, and greater use of endoscopic techniques to remove precancerous lesions (excisional biopsies, then polypectomy, and now endoscopic mucosal resection) all speak to improvements in visualizing and removing precancerous lesions and comfort with colonoscopy as an effective screening tool for preventing IBD-related colorectal cancer.

The remainder of this chapter reviews the latest data and concepts regarding the effectiveness of colonoscopy as a screening tool for colorectal cancer in IBD, recommended screening, and surveillance intervals and techniques (including chromo-endoscopy), as well as how to describe and manage precancerous lesions once found.

Screening Recommendations

Evidence for Screening Programs

Despite endorsement by major societies, no randomized controlled trials have been performed to compare the effectiveness of colonoscopic surveillance compared to no colonoscopic surveillance in reducing the incidence of colorectal cancer and mortality in IBD. However, indirect evidence suggests a benefit to endoscopic surveillance programs in reducing the incidence of CRC in IBD patients [5–9]. As an example, in a small retrospective study, Lutgens et al. demonstrated that IBD patients undergoing regular endoscopic surveillance who were diagnosed with colorectal cancer had improved 5-year CRC survival than those not undergoing surveillance, suggesting a mortality benefit for endoscopic surveillance [5]. Based on these data and extrapolated data showing colonoscopy reduces the incidence and mortality from colorectal cancer in patients without IBD, most societies recommend some form of colonoscopic screening for IBD patients.

Societal Screening and Surveillance Guidelines

Most major gastroenterology societies have developed screening and surveillance guidelines for IBD patients, although some differences exist between guidelines (Table 2.1). It is useful to distinguish the first "screening" exam from the subsequent "surveillance" exams. A summary of United States guidelines suggests that screening colonoscopy should begin in patients 8–10 years after their diagnosis of IBD, should include patients with colon involvement, and be performed at an interval of 1–3 years [10, 11, 15]. Patients who are diagnosed with isolated small bowel Crohn's disease (CD) do not require additional screening beyond that of the average risk individual. Patients with ulcerative colitis (UC) isolated to the rectum do not require subsequent regular surveillance exams after the initial screening exam 8–10 years after diagnosis. Crohn's colitis patients undergoing regular surveillance exams should have one-third or more of the colon involved. Extent of colon involvement should be guided by the greatest extent of endoscopic or histologic involvement of colitis [10]. In patients with primary sclerosing cholangitis (PSC), a screening colonoscopy should be

Table 2.1 Gastrointestinal Society surveillance guidelines [10–14]

Society	First screening colonoscopy	Subsequent colonoscopy interval
American College of Gastroenterology (2010)	All patients 8–10 years after diagnosis Immediately in PSC	Every 1–2 years Every year in PSC
American Gastroenterological Association (2010)	All patients 8–10 years after symptoms onset	Every 1–2 years after screening Every 1–3 years after two negative exams
American Society of Gastrointestinal Endoscopy (2015)	All patients at 8 years after diagnosis with restaging biopsies	Every 1–3 years Lengthen interval after two exams with endoscopically and histologically normal mucosa
British Society of Gastroenterology (2010)	All patients 10 years after diagnosis to determine disease extent and endoscopic risk factors	Yearly in pancolitis with active/moderate inflammation, stricture, PSC, or history of dysplasia or family history of CRC age <50 years Every 3 years in pancolitis with mild inflammation, inflammatory polyps, or family history of CRC >50 years Every 5 years in quiescent pancolitis or left-sided colitis
European Crohn's and Colitis Organization (ECCO) 2017	All patients 8 years after onset of symptoms to assess disease extent and exclude dysplasia Immediately in PSC	Yearly if history of dysplasia or extensive colitis with severe inflammation Every 2–3 years if colitis with mild/moderate inflammation, post-inflammatory polyps, or family history of CRC in first-degree relative Every 5 years for all others

performed at the time of diagnosis of PSC and annually thereafter, given the higher incidence of CRC in these patients.

International guidelines are similar to those from the United States, except that British, European, and Australian guidelines advocate, with limited data, for further risk stratification of patients based on risk for development of colorectal cancer when determining surveillance intervals. These guidelines advocate for repeat colonoscopy every year in patients with high-risk features, every 3 years with intermediate-risk features, and every 5 years with low-risk features [12, 13, 16–20]. Highest-risk patients are considered those with active extensive disease, prior dysplasia, stricture, primary sclerosing cholangitis, or a family history of CRC in a first-degree relative <50 years old [10]. Intermediate-risk patients are those with mild-to-moderate active inflammation, presence of post-inflammatory polyps, or a family history of CRC in a first-degree relative ≥50 years old. Low-risk patients are those without high- and intermediate-risk factors, including those in endoscopic and histologic remissions [13].

Surveillance Technique

An effective screening test must detect the condition at a preclinical and intervenable state that impacts outcome. In the era of fiber-optic technique and then standard-definition colonoscopes, visualization of precancerous lesions (i.e., the preclinical state) was perceived as limited and most dysplasia was considered invisible. To improve the ability to detect these invisible precancerous lesions, surveillance colonoscopy typically involved the performance of four-quadrant biopsies every 10 cm, with the goal of detecting subtle or invisible dysplasia. Over the past decade, application of dye spray (chromoendoscopy) during colonoscopy has been recommended as a way of improving visualization of these subtle lesions by improving the topographic distinction and pit patterns between the inflamed mucosa and precancerous lesions. During this same time, standard-definition (SD) colonoscope technology yielded high-definition (HD) technology, allowing visualization of the mucosa with an even greater level of detail. Today, the question that remains is which of the three screening techniques (high-definition colonoscopy with random biopsy, high-definition chromoendoscopy without random biopsy, high-definition colonoscopy without random biopsy) is sufficient to detect the condition at a preclinical and intervenable state that impacts outcome.

Randomized trials and a meta-analysis of available studies have demonstrated superior dysplasia detection using chromoendoscopy (CE) without random biopsy over standard-definition (SD) white light with random biopsies [21, 22], suggesting superiority of CE over SD white light. A more recent study published in 2017 by Carballal et al. demonstrated superior dysplasia detection using chromoendoscopy without random biopsy technique over SD and HD white light with random biopsies, showing a comparable incremental dysplasia detection yield for CE over SD white light of 51.5% and 52.3% over HD white light [23]. This experience however is not universal. A retrospective study evaluating the use of CE in a real-life setting showed no difference in neoplasia detection rates between CE and white light endoscopy [24]. A randomized controlled trial published in 2018 comparing virtual chromoendoscopy (VC) (using iSCAN Pentax EC-3490Fi with EPKi 7000 Pentax video processor), dye-spray CE, and high-definition white light found that HD white light and VC were non-inferior to dye-spray CE, with the authors concluding that HD white light was sufficient for dysplasia detection [25].

While societal guidelines continue to evolve as new studies are published, Table 2.2 provides a summary of the most current societal statements on the use of random biopsy and chromoendoscopy technique for the surveillance of IBD patients. The American Gastroenterology Association (AGA) statement published in 2010 recommends using a random biopsy strategy of four quadrant biopsies taken every 10 cm for a total of at least 33 biopsies, in addition to targeting suspicious lesions. The statement also supports the use of a chromoendoscopy strategy with targeted biopsies by endoscopists who have expertise in this technique [11]. The Surveillance for Colorectal Endoscopic Neoplasia Detection and Management in IBD Patients International Consensus (SCENIC) statement published in 2015 strongly recommends the use of CE over SD white light (moderate-quality evidence) and suggests the use of CE over HD white light (low-quality evidence). The statement does not recommend the use of virtual chromoendoscopy (use of pseudocolorized electronic image enhancement techniques found in most colonoscopes) as a substitute for dye-spray chromoendoscopy in any situation given multiple studies showing no improvement in dysplasia detection over white light colonoscopy [15]. The American Society of Gastrointestinal Endoscopy (ASGE) 2015 guideline on the role of endoscopy in the IBD patient recommends the use of surface-enhanced chromoendoscopy with resection or targeted biopsy of visible lesions as the preferred surveillance technique [10]. The ASGE endorses the use of the random biopsy technique if chromoendoscopy is not available, or if the yield would be reduced by active inflammation, post-inflammatory polyps, or a poor preparation [10].

Table 2.2 Summary of American Gastrointestinal Societies' Guidelines [10, 11, 15]

Society	Suggested technique
American Gastroenterological Association (2010)	Biopsy-suspicious lesions, four-quadrant biopsies every 10 cm, minimum of 33 random biopsies OR chromoendoscopy
"SCENIC" 2015	High-definition scope recommended over standard definition (strong, low quality) Chromoendoscopy suggested over white light colonoscopy (HD) (conditional/weak, low quality) No specific GRADE recommendation on random biopsies
American Society of Gastrointestinal Endoscopy (2015)	Chromoendoscopy alone is sufficient (no random biopsies); however, consider two biopsies from each segment for histologic staging Random biopsies (four-quadrant, every 10 cm, minimum 33) with targeted biopsies of suspicious lesions as reasonable alternative if chromo not available, significant inflammation, pseudopolyps, or inferior prep

Active inflammation may interfere with visual detection of dysplasia and causes cytologic changes, complicating the pathologist's ability to distinguish inflammation from true dysplasia histologically [26]. Thus, colonoscopic screening and surveillance ideally should be performed when in endoscopic remission [10, 13]. In patients with evidence of active inflammation, medical therapy should be adjusted in an attempt to control inflammation prior to surveillance colonoscopy. This can be achieved in several ways, including escalating or changing therapy or even providing a short steroid taper to control inflammation prior to the examination if there is any concern that inflammation may be contributing to the cytological appearance of dysplasia on biopsies.

Special Topics in Screening

Colonoscopy Preparation

Proper preparation is critical for inspecting the mucosa and detecting dysplasia, particularly flat and slightly raised dysplastic lesions, as residual debris may obscure abnormal areas of the mucosa [26]. Data extrapolated from the general screening population demonstrate that inadequate preparation leads to increased procedure time, lower cecal intubation rates, increased perceived procedure difficulty, early recall for subsequent examinations, and lower polyp detection rate, all negatively impacting the performance of surveillance colonoscopy [27–30].

Compounding the need for meticulous preparation, available data suggests that IBD patients may experience poor tolerance of bowel preparation compared to the general population [31], in addition to having a high rate of risk factors for poor prep such as history of bowel resection [32, 33]. A split-dose regimen of bowel laxative should thus be employed given the ample evidence to date detailing the superiority of a split-dose regimen for achieving adequate bowel preparation in the general population, in addition to improved tolerability and even increasing adenoma detection rates [34–36]. The US Multi-Society Task Force on Colorectal Cancer strongly recommends the use of split-prep cleansing regimens for average risk screening colonoscopy [37], and we extrapolate the recommendation to the IBD community undergoing surveillance colonoscopy.

Chromoendoscopy Technique

Dye-spray chromoendoscopy involves application of a special dye (methylene blue or indigo carmine) onto the mucosa of the colon using either a spray catheter or water jet. Methylene blue, an absorptive dye, is absorbed by non-inflamed mucosa but poorly absorbed by inflamed or dysplastic tissue, thus highlighting potential dysplastic lesions. Indigo carmine, a contrast dye, coats the surface of the colon mucosa, highlighting subtle disruptions of normal contours that indicate dysplastic tissue. Societal statements do not express a preference for either type of dye.

When performing chromoendoscopy, it is important to remember that while application of a dye spray may highlight dysplastic tissue, it is not a substitute for exceptional polyp detection techniques, as findings for dysplasia may still be subtle. Very careful, attentive observation of the colon mucosa should be made, allowing the eye to be drawn to abnormal uptake of the dye spray, being careful not to ignore subtle cues. Besides close inspection, a slow withdrawal can increase the detection of flat dysplasia. A retrospective study from Toruner et al. demonstrated that every additional minute in total colonoscopy time increased the flat dysplasia diagnosis rate by 3.5% ($p = 0.02$) [38].

Chromoendoscopy, although not difficult to learn, does require some training, and videos and reviews on the topic can provide important tips [39]. For example, water lavage on insertion is typically recommended with exchange and application of dye spray reserved for after the cecum is reached. Application of dye spray in a less than properly prepared patient or attempting to clean the colon after the cecum is reached often degrades the quality of the exam or prolongs the procedure. The dye spray is prepared before the procedure. For indigo carmine (0.03%), mix 10 mL of IC 0.8% with 250 mL of water, and for methylene blue (0.04%), mix 10 mL of MB 1% with 240 mL of water.

Once the cecum is intubated, then the dye solution can be attached to the foot pump, exchanging out the sterile water used for insertion or applied using a spray catheter. Examination should take place sequentially of 20–30 cm segments at a time, with re-insertion of the colonoscope to the proximal extent of each segment, followed by careful, slow withdrawal, and inspection of the mucosa. The dye should be applied by directly spraying the antigravity side of the colon lumen, in a circumferential pattern while withdrawing. Suspicious lesions should be inspected more closely using a higher concentration of dye applied to the area (5 mL of IC mixed with 25 mL of water or 10 mL of MB mixed with 40 mL of water) [39]. When learning how to perform chromoendoscopy, a longer block time should be scheduled if possible.

Barriers to Implementing Chromoendoscopy in Practice

Several barriers exist to implementing a chromoendoscopy-based surveillance program for IBD patients. One of these barriers is the perceived notion that CE requires significant expertise to perform. In a 2013 study evaluating dysplasia detection and other endoscopic metrics in endoscopists who were inexperienced in CE, inexperienced endoscopists demonstrated excellent interobserver agreement for identifying dysplastic lesions (kappa score of 0.91 and 0.86 for white light and CE, respectively) [40]. They found dysplasia more often during CE cases (21.3%) versus white light examinations (9.3%), $p = 0.007$. Length of withdrawal time decreased with increasing experience (31 minutes for <5 procedures and 19 minutes for >15 procedures). This study suggests that inexperienced endoscopists can become competent in the CE technique and that most endoscopists have a swift learning curve.

Perceived cost-ineffectiveness may also be a barrier to establishing a CE surveillance program, particularly given the additional procedure time required to perform a high-quality examination. A meta-analysis reported that CE increased procedure time by an average of 11 minutes per procedure [41], but this time may decrease with more experience and if random surveillance biopsies are abandoned in favor of targeted biopsies [42]. There are few studies examining the cost-effectiveness of a CE-based surveillance program, with one study demonstrating cost- effectiveness of CE over white light examinations [43].

Post-inflammatory Polyps

Post-inflammatory polyps (also called pseudopolyps) are considered nonneoplastic lesions arising from the mucosa, likely due to excessive healing following repeated bouts of inflammation and ulceration. They are more commonly found in UC than in CD [44] though estimates in the literature of the prevalence in patients vary significantly, with a recent review demonstrating a prevalence of 53.8% in UC patients and 46.2% in CD patients [45]. The presence of PIPs is thought to be a marker of prior severe inflammatory episodes and may indicate more severe disease. Patients with PIPs are therefore considered to be at a higher risk of colorectal cancer development due to the association with more severe disease [7, 46], with an estimated twofold higher risk in those with previous or present PIPs seen at endoscopy [47–49].

Malignant transformation of PIPs to adenocarcinoma is exceedingly rare, with only two reports of PIPs harboring carcinoma or dysplasia [50, 51]. Overall, the higher risk of colorectal cancer in patients with PIPs is likely due to these patients having more severe, extensive colitis, in addition to the increased challenge of identifying dysplastic lesions in a colon with numerous PIPs present [46, 47]. There is poor interobserver agreement in distinguishing PIPs from dysplastic lesions, with endoscopists without IBD expertise having lower capability to make this distinction [52]. With careful examination of each pseudopolyp, including CE, this distinction should be possible; however, this is limited by the number of PIPs present [53–55]. One study evaluating the nontargeted biopsy approach vs CE in a population with multiple PIPs demonstrated two false-negative results using CE, for which dysplasia was found using the nontargeted approach [41]. For patients with numerous PIPs or in those in whom the diagnosis is not certain, multiple random biopsies should be obtained with repeated examinations. If the number or appearance of PIPs compromises the ability to survey the colon adequately, potential options include referral to a center with expertise in IBD surveillance, vs endoscopic removal of all lesions (if feasible) vs segmental or total colectomy [10,

56–58]. Endoscopic surveillance intervals and techniques should not be altered for those with PIPs in whom endoscopic surveillance is not compromised by the number or size of PIPs, and CE can still be performed in the traditional manner already described in this chapter [10, 12, 13].

Colonic Strictures

The presence of a colonic stricture may also pose challenges for CRC surveillance in IBD. The obvious reason is in the situation that a stricture cannot be traversed, and thus the entire colon cannot be surveyed. The risk of a stricture harboring colorectal cancer in CD is low, and if a stricture can be traversed and biopsied, then repeat endoscopic evaluation is appropriate at a 1-year interval [57]. If the stricture is not traversable, then cross-sectional imaging should be obtained to evaluate the more proximal colon [57]. The exception is if a colonic stricture is found in a patient with CD >20 years, as the concomitant rate of CRC in this population is approximately 12%. Surgical resection should be considered in this situation if surveillance of the whole colon is not possible [57]. Contrary to Crohn's disease, stricture development in a UC patient is a strong indication for colectomy due to the high rate of underlying malignancy [59, 60]. Biopsies, brushings for cytology, and cross-sectional imaging can be considered, with follow-up endoscopy performed in 3–4 months; however, referral to a center with IBD expertise is strongly recommended, and consideration for colectomy is recommended.

When to Stop Surveillance in IBD

Another challenge encountered by endoscopists performing IBD surveillance is when to stop surveying patients with IBD, specifically in the elderly patients. Unfortunately, there is little to no data to guide the decision on when to stop surveillance in IBD patients. The United States Preventive Services Task Force recommends screening until the age of 75 years in the general population, and further screening can be pursued on an individual basis depending on individual characteristics such as life expectancy, medical comorbidities, and history of prior screening [61]. Elderly patients, particularly those 80 years and older, are at a higher risk of complications from colonoscopy, based on studies performed in the general population [62]. The decision on when to stop surveillance in IBD patients needs to be made on an individual basis. Factors to take into account include age, comorbidities, cumulative inflammatory burden, and the presence of concomitant factors such as PSC or prior adenomatous polyps, dysplasia, or malignancy [63]. This decision should be made in a shared decision-making fashion between the patient and their physician [63].

Managing Dysplasia

Modern Terminology for IBD-Related Dysplasia

After identifying a potentially dysplastic area of mucosa, it is of utmost importance to accurately describe the lesion. Important features to describe accurately include where the lesion is, whether it is raised or flat, and whether it is discrete and visible. These descriptors aid in determining the resectability of the lesion and in communicating findings to future endoscopists who may attempt resection or future surveillance. In the past, lesions in IBD patients were described using terms such as dysplasia-associated lesion or mass (DALM), distinguishing it from adenoma-like mass (ALM), which was meant to indicate a sporadic adenoma arising in an area of healthy or noncolitis mucosa. These terms unfortunately are imprecise and led to confusion; therefore, it is currently recommended that these terms be replaced using a modified Paris classification to describe dysplastic lesions found in patients without IBD [15]. The modified classification scheme includes polypoid and nonpolypoid lesions, in addition to a third category, which can be described as "invisible." Invisible lesions should be reserved for those lesions which are truly invisible, meaning that they were identified on random, nontargeted biopsy of the colon mucosa. The Paris classification was further modified to include descriptors for visible dysplasia, including the presence of ulceration and the distinctness of the borders of the lesion (Tables 2.3 and 2.4). This allows for a precise, common language to be used across all screening and surveillance colonoscopies [15, 65].

Table 2.3 Classification for inflammatory bowel disease-associated dysplasia

Term	Definition
Invisible dysplasia	Dysplasia identified on random (nontargeted) biopsies of colon mucosa without a visible lesion
Visible dysplasia	Dysplasia identified on targeted biopsies from a lesion visualized at colonoscopy
Polypoid	Lesion protruding from the mucosa into the lumen ≥2.5 mm
Pedunculated	Lesion attached to the mucosa by a stalk *Paris Classification: Ip*
Sessile	Lesion not attached to the mucosa by a stalk: entire base is contiguous with the mucosa *Paris Classification: Is*
Nonpolypoid	Lesion with little (<2.5 mm) or no protrusion above the mucosa
Superficial elevated	Lesion with protrusion but <2.5 mm above the lumen (less than the height of the closed cup of a biopsy forceps) *Paris Classification: IIa*
Flat	Lesion without protrusion above the mucosa *Paris Classification: IIb*
Depressed	Lesion with at least a portion depressed below the level of the mucosa *Paris Classification: IIc*

Modified from Paris Classification [15, 64]

Table 2.4 Additional characterizations for visible inflammatory bowel disease-associated dysplasia

Feature	Description
Ulcerated	Ulceration (fibrinous-appearing base with depth) within the lesion
Distinct border	Lesion's border is discrete and can be distinguished from surrounding mucosa
Indistinct border	Lesion's border is not discrete and cannot be distinguished from surrounding mucosa

Adapted from SCENIC Consensus Statement [15]

What to Do When Dysplasia Is Identified

Once a potentially dysplastic lesion is identified during colonoscopy, the endoscopist should define it as either polypoid or nonpolypoid and assess the resectability of the lesion, either by the endoscopist or a colleague who is expert in advanced endoscopic resection technique. A potentially resectable lesion should have discrete margins that are identifiable and should appear completely removed on visual inspection following endoscopic resection. Biopsies should be obtained of the tissue surrounding the polyp to ensure that the surrounding tissue is free of dysplasia. If dysplasia is diagnosed on the pathologic specimen, a second expert pathologist should confirm the diagnosis [15]. The histologic exam of the polyp specimen should be consistent with complete removal of the dysplastic lesion [66]. If the lesion is determined to be potentially resectable but will be referred to a colleague who is expert in advanced endoscopic technique, it is important to not attempt a resection as the resultant scarring will make the subsequent resection more challenging. If the lesion is marked with India ink, it should be marked on the wall opposite to the lesion as again the submucosal infiltration of India ink applied adjacent to the lesion can scar the submucosa and make subsequent resection more challenging.

The 2015 SCENIC consensus recommends that in patients with polypoid (i.e., not flat) dysplasia, in whom lesions are completely resected, ongoing surveillance colonoscopy is recommended rather than colectomy [15]. A systematic review of 10 studies including 376 patients with IBD who had polypoid lesions resected reported an annualized risk for CRC of 0.5% over 54 months of follow-up [67]. This recommendation is based on very low-quality evidence, but received a strong recommendation, largely due to what is known about patient views on undergoing colectomy.

In patients with completely resected nonpolypoid (i.e., flat) dysplasia, ongoing surveillance colonoscopy is suggested rather than colectomy. We recommend scheduling follow-up examinations in 3–6 months for those in whom large dysplastic lesions were removed via endoscopic mucosal resection.

Finally, for those patients in whom invisible dysplasia is identified and confirmed via second pathology opinion, referral to an expert in IBD surveillance using chromoendoscopy with high-definition colonoscopy should be made. It is important to note that these specific guidelines are based on very low-quality evidence and are conditional recommendations with the exception of the first one (polypoid lesions) which is a strong recommendation [15].

Future Directions

While the field of CRC surveillance in the IBD patient has come a long way since Crohn and Rosenberg's initial description of malignancy in an IBD patient, there are several identified areas that require more data to refine guidelines and recommendations. For instance, more high-quality data on appropriate surveillance intervals are needed, particularly in the chromoendoscopy era. Further studies should aim to determine the predictive value of a negative CE examination, with a goal toward answering the question of whether a high-quality negative CE examination can reduce the frequency of future interval examinations. Similarly, future directions may include evaluating patients on a more individual basis and tailoring surveillance intervals to patients' risk factors, much like the current European, British, and Australian society guidelines, with a goal of lengthening surveillance intervals for those at lowest risk [12, 13, 17–20]. Biomarker identification and development may also obviate the need for intensive endoscopic surveillance for IBD patients in the future. As already suggested, high-quality data are needed to determine appropriate timing for stopping surveillance in the elderly population to reduce the risks associated with colonoscopy in this population while continuing to mitigate the risk of CRC development. Lastly, efforts will need to be made to overcome the barriers to implementation of CE surveillance programs in the community, including educational interventions, and financial support to undertake these programs.

References

1. Lopez A, Collet-Fenetrier B, Belle A, Peyrin-Biroulet L. Patients' knowledge and fear of colorectal cancer risk in inflammatory bowel disease. J Dig Dis. 2016;17(6):383–91.
2. Crohn BB, Rosenberg H. The sigmoidoscopic pictureof chronic ulcerative colitis (nonspecific). Am J Med Sci. 1925;170:220–8.
3. Warren S, Sommers SC. Cicatrizing enteritis (regional ileitis) as a pathologic entity. Am J Pathol. 1948;24:475–501.
4. Jones JH. Colonic cancer and Crohn's disease. Gut. 1969;10:651–4.
5. Lutgens MW, Oldenburg B, Siersema PD, van Bodegraven AA, Dijkstra G, Hommes DW, et al. Colonoscopic surveillance improves survival after colorectal cancer diagnosis in inflammatory bowel disease. Br J Cancer. 2009;101(10):1671–5.
6. Choi PM, Nugent FW, Schoetz DJ Jr, et al. Colonoscopic surveillance reduces mortality from colorectal cancer in ulcerative colitis. Gastroenterology. 1993;105:418–24.
7. Eaden J, Abrams K, Ekbom A, et al. Colorectal cancer prevention in ulcerative colitis: a case-control study. Aliment Pharmacol Ther. 2000;14:145–53.
8. Karlen P, Kornfeld D, Brostrom O, et al. Is colonoscopic surveillance reducing colorectal cancer mortality in ulcerative colitis? A population based case control study. Gut. 1998;42:711–4.

9. Lashner BA, Kane SV, Hanauer SB. Colon cancer surveillance in chronic ulcerative colitis: a historical cohort study. Am J Gastroenterol. 1990;85:1083–7.
10. American Society for Gastrointestinal Endoscopy Standards of Practice Committee, Shergill AK, Lightdale JR, Bruining DH, Acosta RD, Chandrasekhara V, et al. The role of endoscopy in inflammatory bowel disease. Gastrointest Endosc. 2015;81(5):1101–21.e1–13.
11. Farraye FA, Odze RD, Eaden J, Itzkowitz SH, McCabe RP, Dassopoulos T, et al. AGA medical position statement on the diagnosis and management of colorectal neoplasia in inflammatory bowel disease. Gastroenterology. 2010;138(2):738–45.
12. Cairns SR, Scholefield JH, Steele RJ, Dunlop MG, Thomas HJ, Evans GD, et al. Guidelines for colorectal cancer screening and surveillance in moderate and high risk groups (update from 2002). Gut. 2010;59(5):666–89.
13. Annese V, Daperno M, Rutter MD, et al. European evidence based consensus for endoscopy in inflammatory bowel disease. J Crohn's Colitis. 2013;7:982–1018.
14. Kornbluth A, Sachar DB, Practice Parameters Committee of the American College of Gastroenterology. Ulcerative colitis practice guidelines in adults: American College of Gastroenterology, Practice Parameters Committee. Am J Gastroenterol. 2010;105(3):501–23; quiz 24.
15. SCENIC international consensus statement on surveillance and management of dysplasia in inflammatory bowel disease. Gastrointest Endosc. 2015;81(3):489–501.
16. Mowat C, Cole A, Windsor A, et al. Guidelines on the management of inflammatory bowel disease in adults. Gut. 2011;60:571–607.
17. Howdle P, Wendy A, Rutter M. Colonoscopic surveillance for prevention of colorectal cancer in people with ulcerative colitis, Crohn's disease or adenomas. National Institute for Health and Clinical Excellence (NICE) Clinical guideline. National Institutes of Health and Clinical Excellence;118. London: National Institute for Health and Clinical Excellence; 2011.
18. Party CCACSW, editor. Clinical Practice Guidelines for Surveillance Colonoscopy in adenoma follow-up; following curative resection of colorectal cancer; and for cancer surveillance in inflammatory bowel disease. Sydney: Cancer Council of Australia; 2011.
19. Van Assche G, Dignass A, Bokemeyer B, Danese S, Gionchetti P, Moser G, et al. Second European evidence-based consensus on the diagnosis and management of ulcerative colitis part 3: special situations. J Crohns Colitis. 2013;7(1):1–33.
20. Kaminski MF, Hassan C, Bisschops R, et al. Advanced imaging for detection and differentiation of colorectal neoplasia: European Society of Gastrointestinal Endoscopy (ESGE) guideline. Endoscopy. 2014;46(05):435–57.
21. Iannone A, Ruospo M, Wong G, Principi M, Barone M, Strippoli GFM, et al. Chromoendoscopy for surveillance in ulcerative colitis and Crohn's disease: a systematic review of randomized trials. Clin Gastroenterol Hepatol. 2017;15(11):1684–97.e11.
22. Soetikno R, Subramanian V, Kaltenbach T, Rouse RV, Sanduleanu S, Suzuki N, et al. The detection of nonpolypoid (flat and depressed) colorectal neoplasms in patients with inflammatory bowel disease. Gastroenterology. 2013;144(7):1349–52, 52.e1–6.
23. Carballal S, Maisterra S, Lopez-Serrano A, Gimeno-Garcia AZ, Vera MI, Marin-Garbriel JC, et al. Real-life chromoendoscopy for neoplasia detection and characterisation in long-standing IBD. Gut. 2018;67(1):70–8.
24. Mooiweer E, van der Meulen-de Jong AE, Ponsioen CY, Fidder HH, Siersema PD, Dekker E, et al. Chromoendoscopy for surveillance in inflammatory bowel disease does not increase neoplasia detection compared with conventional colonoscopy with random biopsies: results from a large retrospective study. Am J Gastroenterol. 2015;110(7):1014–21.
25. Iacucci M, Kaplan GG, Panaccione R, Akinola O, Lethebe BC, Lowerison M, et al. A randomized trial comparing high definition colonoscopy alone with high definition dye spraying and electronic virtual chromoendoscopy for detection of colonic neoplastic lesions during IBD surveillance colonoscopy. Am J Gastroenterol. 2018;113(2):225–34.
26. Nett A, Velayos F, McQuaid K. Quality bowel preparation for surveillance colonoscopy in patients with inflammatory bowel disease is a must. Gastrointest Endosc Clin N Am. 2014;24(3):379–92.

27. Harewood GC, Sharma VK, de Garmo P. Impact of colonoscopy preparation quality on detection of suspected colonic neoplasia. Gastrointest Endosc. 2003;58(1):76–9.
28. Rex DK, Imperiale TF, Latinovich DR, Bratcher LL. Impact of bowel preparation on efficiency and cost of colonoscopy. Am J Gastroenterol. 2002;97(7):1696–700.
29. Froehlich F, Wietlisbach V, Gonvers J-J, et al. Impact of colonic cleansing on quality and diagnostic yield of colonoscopy_the European Panel of Appropriateness of Gastrointestinal Endoscopy European multicenter study. Gastrointest Endosc. 2005;61(3):378–84.
30. Parra-Blanco A, Nicolas-Perez D, Gimeno-Garcia A, et al. The timing of bowel preparation before colonoscopy determines the quality of cleansing, and is a significant factor contributing to the detection of flat lesions: a randomized study. World J Gastroenterol. 2006;12(38):6161–6.
31. Bessissow T, Van Keerberghen C-A, Van Oudenhove L, et al. Anxiety is associated with impaired tolerance of colonoscopy preparation in inflammatory bowel disease and controls. J Crohn's Colitis. 2013;7(11):e580–e7.
32. Lim SW, Seo YW, Sinn DH, et al. Impact of previous gastric or colonic resection on polyethylene glycol bowel preparation for colonoscopy. Surg Endosc. 2012;26:1554–9.
33. Chung YW, Han DS, Park KH, et al. Patient factors predictive of inadequate bowel preparation using polyethylene glycol. J Clin Gastroenterol. 2009;43:448–52.
34. Kilgore TW, Abdinoor AA, Szary NM, et al. Bowel preparation with split-dose polyethylene glycol before colonoscopy: a meta-analysis of randomized controlled trials. Gastrointest Endosc. 2011;73(6):1240–5.
35. Enestvedt BK, Tofani C, Laine LA, Tierney A, Fennerty MB. 4-Liter split-dose polyethylene glycol is superior to other bowel preparations, based on systematic review and meta-analysis. Clin Gastroenterol Hepatol. 2012;10(11):1225–31.
36. Gurudu SR, Ramirez FC, Harrison ME, et al. Increased adenoma detection rate with system-wide implementation of a split-dose preparation for colonoscopy. Gastrointest Endosc. 2012;76:603–8.
37. Johnson DA, Barkun AN, Cohen LB, Dominitz JA, Kaltenbach T, Martel M, et al. Optimizing adequacy of bowel cleansing for colonoscopy: recommendations from the US Multi-Society Task Force on Colorectal Cancer. Am J Gastroenterol. 2014;109(10):1528–45.
38. Toruner M, Harewood GC, Loftus EV Jr, et al. Endoscopic factors in the diagnosis of colorectal dysplasia in chronic inflammatory bowel disease. Inflamm Bowel Dis. 2005;11(5):428–34.
39. Sanduleanu S, Kaltenbach T, Barkun A, McCabe RP, Velayos F, Picco MF, et al. A roadmap to the implementation of chromoendoscopy in inflammatory bowel disease colonoscopy surveillance practice. Gastrointest Endosc. 2016;83(1):213–22.
40. Picco MF, Pasha S, Leighton JA, Bruining D, Loftus EV, Thomas CS, et al. Procedure time and the determination of polypoid abnormalities with experience. Inflamm Bowel Dis. 2013;19:1913–20.
41. Kiesslich R, Fritsch J, Holtmann M, Koehler HH, Stolte M, Kanzler S, et al. Methylene blue-aided chromoendoscopy for the detection of intraepithelial neoplasia and colon cancer in ulcerative colitis. Gastroenterology. 2003;124(4):880–8.
42. Leong RW, Butcher RO, Picco MF. Implementation of image-enhanced endoscopy into solo and group practices for dysplasia detection in Crohn's disease and ulcerative colitis. Gastrointest Endosc Clin N Am. 2014;24(3):419–25.
43. Konijeti GG, Shrime MG, Ananthakrishnan AN, Chan AT. Cost effectiveness analysis of chromoendsocopy for colorectal cacner surveillance in patients with ulcerative colitis. Gastrointest Endosc. 2014;79:455–65.
44. Margulis AR, Goldberg HI, Lawson TL, et al. The overlapping spectrum of ulcerative and granulomatous colitis: a roentgenographic-pathologic study. Am J Roentgenol Radium Therapy, Nucl Med. 1971;113:325–34.
45. Maggs JR, Browning LC, Warren BF, Travis SP. Obstructing giant post-inflammatory polyposis in ulcerative colitis: case report and review of the literature. J Crohns Colitis. 2008;2(2):170–80.
46. De Dombal FT, Watts JM, Watkinson G, Goligher JC. Local complications of ulcerative colitis: stricture, pseudopolyposis, and carcinoma of the colon and rectum. Br Med J. 1966;1:1442–7.

47. Velayos FS, Loftus EV Jr, Jess T, Harmsen WS, Bida J, Zinsmeister AR, et al. Predictive and protective factors associated with colorectal cancer in ulcerative colitis: a case-control study. Gastroenterology. 2006;130(7):1941–9.

48. Rutter MD, Saunders BP, Wilkinson KH, Rumbles S, Schofield G, Kamm MA, et al. Cancer surveillance in longstanding ulcerative colitis: endoscopic appearances help predict cancer risk. Gut. 2004;53(12):1813–6.

49. Baars JE, Looman CWN, Steyerberg EW, Beukers R, Tan ACITL, Weusten BLAM, et al. The risk of inflammatory bowel disease-related colorectal carcinoma is limited: results from a nationwide nested case–control study. Am J Gastroenterol. 2010;106(2):319–28.

50. Dukes CE. The surgical pathology of ulcerative colitis. Ann R Coll Surg Engl. 1954;14:389–400.

51. Kusunoki M, Nishigami T, Yanagi H, et al. Occult cancer localized in giant pseudopolyposis. Am J Gastroenterol. 1992;87(3):379–81.

52. Farraye FA, Waye JD, Moscandrew M, Heeren TC, Odze RD. Variability in the diagnosis and management of adenoma-like and non-adenoma-like dysplasia-associated lesions or masses in inflammatory bowel disease: an Internet-based study. Gastrointest Endosc. 2007;66(3):519–29.

53. Kudo S-E, Tamura S, Nakajima T, et al. Diagnosis of colorectal tumorous lesions by magnifying endoscopy. Gastrointest Endosc. 1996;44(1):8–14.

54. Koinuma K, Togashi K, Konishi F, Kirii Y, Horie H, Okada M, et al. Localized giant inflammatory polyposis of the cecum associated with distal ulcerative colitis. J Gastroenterol. 2003;38(9):880–3.

55. Bernstein CN. The color of dysplasia in ulcerative colitis. Gastroenterology. 2003;124:1135–49.

56. Choi YS, Suh JP, Lee IT, Kim JK, Lee SH, Cho KR, et al. Regression of giant pseudopolyps in inflammatory bowel disease. J Crohns Colitis. 2012;6(2):240–3.

57. Itzkowitz SH, Present DH. Consensus conference: colorectal cancer screening and surveillance in inflammatory bowel disease. Inflamm Bowel Dis. 2005;11:314–21.

58. Itzkowitz SH, Harpaz N. Diagnosis and management of dysplasia in patients with inflammatory bowel diseases. Gastroenterology. 2004;126(6):1634–48.

59. Gumaste V, Sachar DB, Greenstein AJ. Benign and malignant colorectal strictures in ulcerative colitis. Gut. 1992;33:938–41.

60. Reiser JR, Waye JD, Janowitz HD, Harpaz N. Adenocarcinoma in strictures of ulcerative colitis without antecedent dysplasia by colonoscopy. Am J Gastroenterol. 1994;89(1):119–22.

61. Rex DK, Boland CR, Dominitz JA, Giardiello FM, Johnson DA, Kaltenbach T, et al. Colorectal cancer screening: recommendations for physicians and patients from the U.S. Multi-Society Task Force on Colorectal Cancer. Am J Gastroenterol. 2017;112(7):1016–30.

62. Day LW, Kwon A, Inadomi JM, Walter LC, Somsouk M. Adverse events in older patients undergoing colonoscopy: a systematic review and meta-analysis. Gastrointest Endosc. 2011;74(4):885–96.

63. Long MD, Sands BE. When do you start and when do you stop screening for colon cancer in inflammatory bowel disease? Clin Gastroenterol Hepatol. 2018;16(5):621–3.

64. The Paris classification of superficial neoplastic lesions: esophagus, stomach, and colon. Gastrointest Endosc. 2003;58(suppl):53–43.

65. Velayos F, Kathpalia P, Finlayson E. Changing paradigms in detection of dysplasia and management of patients with inflammatory bowel disease: is colectomy still necessary? Gastroenterology. 2017;152(2):440–50 e1.

66. Kaltenbach T, Sandborn WJ. Endoscopy in inflammatory bowel disease: advances in dysplasia detection and management. Gastrointest Endosc. 2017;86(6):962–71.

67. Wanders LK, Dekker E, Pullens B, Bassett P, Travis SP, East JE. Cancer risk after resection of polypoid dysplasia in patients with longstanding ulcerative colitis: a meta-analysis. Clin Gastroenterol Hepatol. 2014;12(5):756–64.

Chapter 3
Skin Cancer Risk and Screening in Patients with Inflammatory Bowel Disease

Reid L. Hopkins, Jamie Abbott, Debjani Sahni, and Francis A. Farraye

Introduction

The most common skin cancers are melanoma and non-melanoma skin cancer, the latter a group that includes basal cell carcinoma (BCC) and cutaneous squamous cell carcinoma (SCC). Melanoma is notorious for a high metastatic potential with low 5-year survival when diagnosed at an advanced stage. Non-melanoma skin cancers (NMSC), on the other hand, have a much lower metastatic potential as well as low overall mortality. However, by virtue of being by far the most common cancer group in the United States, annual spending for NMSC makes it among the most costly cancers within the Medicare population [1, 2]. While there are numerous dermatologic manifestations of inflammatory bowel disease, it has become more apparent in the past two decades, especially as the use of immunomodulators and biologics has grown, that skin cancer is an important risk in IBD.

Experience in solid organ transplant has firmly established that a complication of long-term immunosuppression is an increased risk of the development of NMSC, especially squamous cell carcinoma. In this population, the incidence of SCC is markedly increased, up to 65–250 times the general population while the incidence of BCC is about tenfold that of the general population [3]. In addition to being more common, SCC is more aggressive in this population with more rapid growth, higher recurrence rates, and increased risk of metastasis. Finally, it has been well

R. L. Hopkins · F. A. Farraye (✉)
Section of Gastroenterology, Boston Medical Center, Boston University School of Medicine, Boston, MA, USA
e-mail: reid.hopkins@bmc.org; francis.farraye@bmc.org

J. Abbott · D. Sahni
Department of Dermatology, Boston Medical Center, Boston University School of Medicine, Boston, MA, USA
e-mail: jamie.abbott@bmc.org; debjani.Sahni@bmc.org

© Springer Nature Switzerland AG 2019
J. D. Feuerstein, A. S. Cheifetz (eds.), *Cancer Screening in Inflammatory Bowel Disease*, https://doi.org/10.1007/978-3-030-15301-4_3

demonstrated that cumulative dose of immunosuppressants is associated with increased risk of development of SCC in a dose-dependent fashion [4].

These alarming findings spurred research into the impact of the immunosuppressants used in the treatment of IBD on the risk of skin cancer. The sum of evidence now suggests that patients with IBD, somewhat surprisingly, have an increased risk of developing melanoma, independent of medication exposure, in addition to an increased risk of NMSC, especially in the setting of thiopurine exposure. Whether TNFα inhibitors or other newer biologics affect the incidence or natural history of melanoma is uncertain. These findings have led to management guidelines that recommend sun exposure precautions and skin cancer screening, though optimal strategies for the latter have yet to be fully defined. This chapter will review the literature in this field to inform a rational approach to management and prevention of skin cancer in the IBD patient.

Epidemiology of Skin Cancer in the United States

While there are many different cancers of the skin, for the purposes of this chapter, we will focus on the most common types: BCC, cutaneous SCC, and melanoma. All are epidermal in origin, with the rare exception of melanomas arising in the eyes, central nervous system, oral mucosa, and intestines [5, 6].

Non-melanoma Skin Cancer

Basal cell and squamous cell carcinomas are often grouped together under the umbrella term, non-melanoma skin cancer (NMSC) or keratinocyte carcinomas [7]. This delineation can be a useful simplification due to the very different prognoses and management recommendations the term implies when compared to a diagnosis of melanoma.

Basal cell carcinoma is a cancer of the progenitor keratinocyte cells located in the stratum basale of the epidermis. Typical BCCs are most common on the head and neck and can appear as pearly papules with rolled borders and arborizing telangiectasias (Fig. 3.1). Some have pigments or can ulcerate. Patients often complain of a slow growing lesion or a new spot that fails to heal. The lesions may be asymptomatic or cause intermittent bleeding or pruritus [7]. The most common BCC subtype is nodular (50–80%), followed by superficial (10–30%) [7, 8]. Other rarer subtypes include morpheaform, infundibulocystic, fibroepithelial, and infiltrative [8]. Each subtype is histologically distinct and has some bearing on the clinical appearance and behavior of the lesion [7]. That being said, a single lesion can exhibit features of multiple subtypes on histology [8].

Research suggests that the development of BCC is primarily associated with an intermittent, acute ultraviolet light exposure, as in the case of blistering sunburns

Fig. 3.1 Basal cell carcinoma

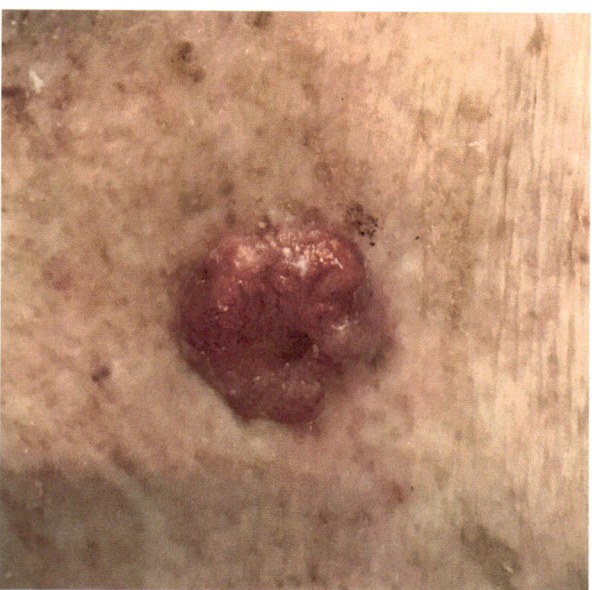

Table 3.1 Risk factors for melanoma and NMSC

Risk factors
History of UV light exposure
Increased age (more relevant in NMSC)
Fair skin
Male gender
Immune suppression
Family history and certain genetic disorders
Ionizing radiation, chronic wounds, burns, scars (NMSC)
Multiple melanocytic nevi (melanoma)

[9]. There is data to suggest that cumulative sun exposure over time also poses an increased risk [10, 11]. It is important to remember that tanning beds and phototherapy are other sources of UV to which patients may have been exposed. Age is an important risk factor, with incidence doubling between the ages of 40 and 70 [12]. Other risk factors include male gender, fair skin, certain genetic disorders, like nevoid basal cell carcinoma syndrome, and immune suppression [7]. Table 3.1 summarizes risk factors for the subtypes of skin cancer.

Cutaneous squamous cell carcinoma is a cancer of the squamous cells normally located in the epidermis. The lesions of squamous cell carcinoma most commonly appear on sun-exposed areas as ill-defined pink, rough, or scaly macules or papules (Fig. 3.2). Small dotted vessels and glomerular vessels can be identified on dermoscopy [13]. SCCs can also arise in chronic wounds, burns, or otherwise damaged skin, where they can be harder to detect without a high index of suspicion [14]. Histologically, SCCs range from well to poorly differentiated, with poorly differentiated SCCs having a worse prognosis [15]. The SCC subtypes with the

Fig. 3.2 Squamous cell
carcinoma

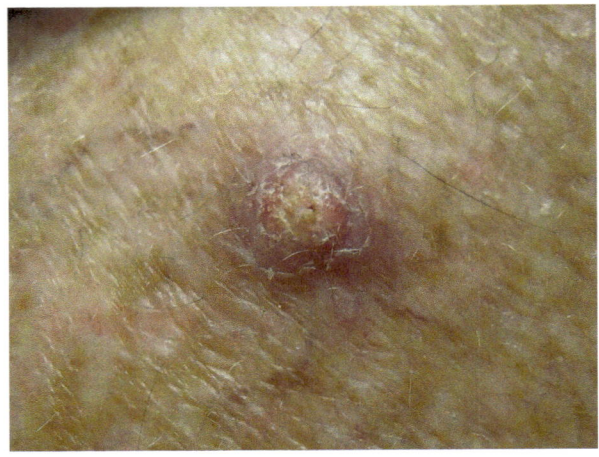

worst prognoses are the desmoplastic and adenosquamous variants which boast
both a higher rate of recurrence and metastasis compared to other variants of SCC
[16, 17].

The development of SCC is related to a history of childhood sunburns and
cumulative sun exposure [9, 18]. Patients with a history of actinic keratoses (AK)
have been shown to be more likely to develop SCC, and AKs are often used as a
clinical marker of sun exposure and risk for the development of SCC [19].
Periungual and anogenital SCC are associated with human papilloma virus and are
not thought to be related to sun exposure given their sun-protected locations [20].
Age is also a risk factor in the development of SCC, with onset most common in the
sixth decade [21]. Other risk factors include fair skin, male gender (3:1 male-to-
female ratio), exposure to certain compounds (arsenic, polycyclic aromatic hydro-
carbons, nitrosamines, and alkylating agents), exposure to ionizing radiation, and
immunosuppression [14, 22, 23]. The immunosuppressed state following solid
organ transplant increases the risk of developing an SCC by 65–250 times depending on the level of immune suppression [24–26]. Similarly, the immune dysregula-
tion in chronic lymphocytic leukemia (CLL) confers an 8–10 times increased risk
[27–29].

Different studies have quoted basal cell carcinomas as making up 50–80% of
non-melanoma skin cancers, while cutaneous squamous cell carcinomas account
for 20–50% [1, 30, 31]. Though the exact incidence of non-melanoma skin cancer
in the United States is not known due to the lack of inclusion of these diagnoses in
the US tumor registries, it is widely understood that non-melanoma skin cancer is
the most commonly diagnosed cancer in the United States [32, 33]. In 1996, it was
estimated that one in five people will develop a skin cancer in the United States,
with at least 97% of these being NMSC [34]. More recently, in 2012, it was estimated that there were over five million cases of NMSC in the United States [1]. The
incidence in the United States rises by an estimated 4–8% yearly [32]. The incidence of metastatic BCC is estimated at 0.0028–0.55%, and deaths from BCCs are

incredibly rare [35, 36]. SCC, on the other hand, is associated with more significant mortality than that associated with BCC, though overall remains low compared to mortality from most other types of cancers. Data from Karia et al. estimates that between 3932 and 8791 Americans died from SCC in 2012 [37]. A different study of patients in Rhode Island reported age-adjusted mortality from nongenital SCC as 0.26/100,000 [36].

Although mortality from NMSC is relatively low compared to most other cancers, the impact of this diagnosis should not be ignored. Beyond the potentially deforming effects of treatment, the average annual cost of treating non-melanoma skin cancers in the US has increased by 126.2% between 2002–2006 and 2007–2011, reflecting an increase from 3.6 to 8.1 billion US dollars [38]. When compared to other types of cancers, for which the cost of treatment has only increased by 25.1% on average, it is clear that controlling costs will become increasingly more vital in sustaining healthcare delivery for skin cancers [38].

Melanoma

Melanoma is a cancer of melanocytes, the pigment-producing cells, primarily located in the basal layer of the epidermis. The lesions of melanoma are often characterized as changing, asymmetric, irregular pigmented macules, papules, or nodules containing multiple different colors (Fig. 3.3). They can sometimes be particularly challenging to diagnose, however, as they can also be small, innocuous appearing, and can lack pigment entirely, as in amelanotic melanoma. There are many different types of primary melanoma including superficial spreading, nodular, lentigo maligna, and acral lentiginous melanoma. In addition to these and to amelanotic melanoma, other types include melanoma with features of Spitz nevus, desmoplastic melanoma, and ocular and mucosal melanomas [6, 39].

Fig. 3.3 Melanoma

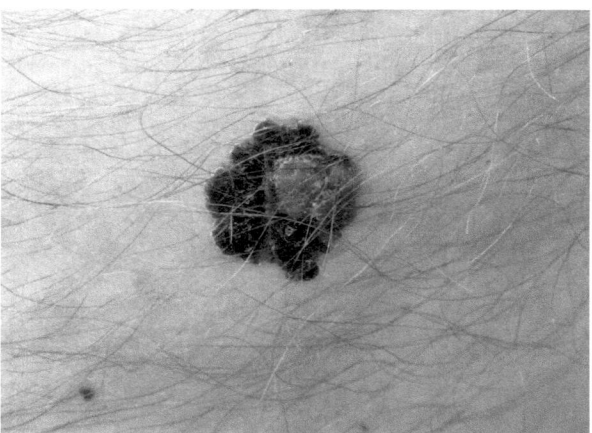

Fair skin, sunburning easily, having red or blonde hair, blue eyes, and male gender are the risk factors for the development of melanoma [40–43]. In men, the most common location is the trunk, while in women it is the lower extremities [41]. The average age of diagnosis in the United States is slightly younger than that of NMSC, ranging from 54 to 64 years of age [40].

An intermittent intense exposure to UV light is an important risk factor in the development of melanoma [41, 44]. Tanning beds have been a contributing factor to the development of melanomas, especially in young women. In a cohort studied in Minnesota, women under 30 who had used tanning beds were six times more likely to develop melanoma when compared to their age-matched peers [45]. Additionally, increased numbers of melanocytic nevi, even those that are clinically normal-appearing are associated, nearly linearly, with an increased risk of melanoma [46]. Similarly, the presence of five or more atypical nevi on exam confers a tenfold increased risk [46].

Genetic factors have also been identified. One of the genes implicated in the increased risk of melanoma is CDKN2A/p16. This gene is of particular clinical importance, as mutations therein confer a 20% risk of pancreatic cancer as well [47]. Multiple genetic syndromes with an associated increased risk of melanoma have been described. The details of these syndromes are beyond the scope of this chapter. The authors recommend *The Melanoma Handbook* by Stephan Ariyan and Harriet Klugar and the chapters pertaining to melanoma in *Dermatology* by Jean Bolognia, should the reader wish to learn more [48, 49].

The National Cancer Institute SEER program ranks melanoma as the sixth most common cancer and the fifth most common in men in the United States [40]. Over the past 30 years, melanoma rates have increased by three times in lighter skinned individuals in both the United States and Europe [41]. It is currently estimated that roughly 2.3% of people in the United States will be diagnosed in their lifetimes [40]. By these standards alone, melanoma is an extremely common cancer in the United States, and though it is not as common as the non-melanoma skin cancers, its prognosis is far worse. The 10-year survival of a patient with visceral disease is only 10–15% [42].

While in the last several years, mortality rates in the United States have steadied, previous estimations have indicated that one person dies from melanoma in the United States every 60 min [50]. Mortality depends on both the stage of the melanoma and other factors, like age, race, gender, and immune status [42, 51]. Women and patients younger than 65 tend to have a better prognosis. Patients with an intact immune system fair better than the immunocompromised ones [42]. The Breslow depth, which is the tumor thickness measured vertically on histology, and the presence or absence of ulceration are the most impactful prognostic factors with thicker, ulcerated tumors having a worse prognosis [41, 52].

With regard to both SCC and melanoma, darker-skinned individuals are less likely to develop these cancers than fair-skinned individuals, but demonstrate poorer prognoses when diagnosed [53–55].

Epidemiology of Skin Cancer in IBD

Multiple population-based studies and meta-analyses have examined the epidemiology of skin cancer in the IBD population. Ekbom and colleagues were among the first to report an association between IBD and the development of squamous cell carcinoma [56]. Their data came from a population-based cohort from Sweden including 4776 patients who were diagnosed with IBD between 1958 and 1984. They noted an increased incidence of SCC in all patients with IBD (standardized incidence ratio [SIR] 2.2; 95% CI 1.1–3.9); the excess incidence was most notable in the Crohn's disease subpopulation (SIR 5.5; 95% CI 2–11.9) with no significant difference in the ulcerative colitis population. Jess and colleagues looked at a smaller population cohort with CD in Copenhagen County in Denmark ($n = 374$) and found an increased incidence of melanoma and SCC (standardized morbidity ratio of 2.03 and 1.61, respectively), though their absolute numbers of cases were low and the association failed to reach statistical significance [57]. On the other hand, in a Canadian matched cohort study in Manitoba with 5529 IBD cases matched 1:10 to controls, there was no significant difference in the incidence of melanoma in the IBD population [58]. NMSC was not reported on in this study.

Given these variable results, a meta-analysis in 2010 examined the incidence of extraintestinal cancers in the IBD population in eight population-based studies with a total pooled population of 17,052 patients [59]. They found a significantly elevated pooled standardized incidence ratio (SIR) of 1.79 (95% CI 1.01–3.16) for squamous cell carcinoma among all patients with IBD. This was largely driven by patients with Crohn's disease where the SIR was 2.35 (95% CI 1.43–3.86). The SIR for patients with ulcerative colitis trended toward, but did not reach, statistical significance (SIR 1.68; 95% CI 0.9–3.12). The pooled SIR for melanoma in undifferentiated IBD patients, on the other hand, was not significantly elevated (1.17, 95% CI 0.66–2.08). The majority of the included populations were European, but two studies did examine populations in Canada and in Minnesota. The association with immunosuppressive medication or other potential risk factors was not included in their analysis. Another large population study was added to the literature in 2014 [60]. The authors used Danish healthcare databases to examine patients diagnosed with CD or UC between 1978 and 2010 and followed them until the incidence of cancer, death, or emigration. The study examined 13,756 patients with CD and 35,152 patients with UC and found significant association between IBD and NMSC with the SIRs of 2.1 (1.8–2.3) for CD and 1.8 (1.7–2) for UC. There was a suggestion of an association between melanoma and IBD, but this association did not reach significance (SIR of 1.4 [1–1.9] for CD and 1.1 [0.9–1.3] for UC).

Other more recent studies have shown an association between melanoma and IBD. In a large ($n = 108,579$ patients with IBD) retrospective case–control study using a large health claims database in the United States, Long and colleagues found an association between melanoma and IBD with an incidence rate ratio (IRR) of 1.29 (95% CI 1.09–1.53) [61]. An alarming finding in this study was an association in a nested case-control analysis between therapy with biologics and development of melanoma with an odds ratio of 1.88 (95% CI 1.08–3.29). Since this study included data prior to 2009, biologic exposure in their population was essentially only TNFα inhibitors. Similarly, a more recent meta-analysis confirmed an association between IBD and melanoma [62]. These authors examined 12 cohort studies comprising 172,837 patients and found a crude incidence ratio of melanoma of 27.5 cases/100,000 person-years. They found IBD to be associated with a 37% increase in risk of melanoma (RR, 1.37; 95% CI 1.10–1.70). Interestingly, melanoma risk was elevated (RR 1.52; 95% CI 1.02–2.25) in the IBD population prior to the introduction of biologics (1998) in this analysis but not after (RR 1.08; 95% CI 0.59–1.96), though there were fewer studies included in the latter group. These two studies together suggest an increased risk of melanoma in IBD patients perhaps irrespective of specific therapeutic exposure.

In meta-analyses, then, IBD has been associated with an increased risk of both non-melanoma skin cancer and melanoma. Several studies have evaluated further risk stratification within the IBD population based on IBD type and medication exposure. This will be the focus of the further sections in this chapter.

Risk Factors Within the IBD Population

Patients can be further stratified for the development of skin cancer based on known risk factors. Risk factors for skin cancer among the general population have been well described in the above sections and presumably apply in the IBD population. In addition, an understanding of the current evidence for the role of medications and IBD-subtype disease-specific risk factors is critical for the practicing gastroenterologist.

Thiopurines and Skin Cancer

As noted above, IBD itself appears to be a risk factor for the development of both categories of skin cancer. The reason for this increased risk of both NMSC and melanoma in IBD patients is complex with several contributing factors. As noted in the introduction, the risk of squamous cell carcinoma in the post-transplant population is well recognized, pointing to immunosuppression as an implicated exposure. Indeed, one study showed that in human cell lines, six thioguanine (6-TG, an azathioprine metabolite) accumulates in cell DNA and is susceptible to ultraviolet A (UVA) radiation at physiologic doses [63]. When exposed to UVA, the major component of solar radiation, 6-TG, generates reactive oxygen species, which in turn lead to the accumulation of DNA mutations, a potential precursor to carcinogenesis. The same group showed the clinical relevance of these in vitro findings in another study [64]. They measured minimal erythema dose (MED) after exposure to UVA before and after 12 weeks of therapy in human subjects with azathioprine and showed significant skin sensitization to UVA exposure after treatment. Biopsies of treated patients also showed increased 6-TG in cells. These findings provide a biologically plausible mechanism for the role of thiopurines in the development of squamous cell carcinoma. In addition, there is evidence that azathioprine is associated with mutations of the tumor suppressor PTCH gene in basal cell carcinomas [65].

Large studies have confirmed the clinical relevance of these in vitro findings. The CESAME cohort in France enrolled 19,486 patients with IBD prospectively between May 2004 and June 2005 and followed them through December 31, 2007, recording baseline data, immunosuppression regimen, and incidence of cancer during follow-up [66]. This cohort showed a standardized incidence ratio (SIR) for development of NMSC of 2.89 in all patients with IBD. The SIR for patients with ongoing thiopurine use was notably higher at 7.06 and past thiopurine exposure was 5.19. In patients without thiopurine exposure, the rate of NMSC development was similar to the general population. This finding persisted in multivariate analysis with a hazard ratio of 5.9 for ongoing thiopurine treatment and 3.9 for past thiopurine exposure. Of note, for consideration in developing screening strategies, the excess risk of development of NMSC was observed even in the population younger than 50 years old. The same authors found no association in their data set between melanoma and IBD or melanoma and thiopurines. The number of patients exposed to biologics was too small to analyze in this study. This study also did not collect data on dose and duration of thiopurine exposure. Regardless, this landmark study provided rich, prospective data that can be used to provide patients with accurate risk information.

In another landmark study, the association between thiopurine exposure and the development of skin cancer was examined in the VA population in a retrospective cohort with data collected between 2001 and 2011 [67]. The authors adjusted for demographics, UV radiation exposure, and healthcare utilization. The adjusted hazard ratio of developing NMSC while on thiopurine was 2.1 ($P < 0.0001$) and 0.7 ($p = 0.07$) after stopping, implying unlike the previous studies described above that risk goes back to baseline after discontinuation. Compellingly, and consistent with findings in the post-transplant population, the incidence rate of NMSC among those who never used thiopurines was 3.7 compared with 5.8, 7.9, 8.3, 7.8, and 13.6 per 1000 person-years for the 1st, 2nd, 3th, 4th, and 5th year of thiopurine use, respectively.

Finally, a meta-analysis pooled 8 studies totaling 60,351 patients and found a pooled adjusted hazards ratio of developing NMSC after exposure to thiopurines in IBD patients of 2.28 (95% CI 1.5–3.45) [68]. This study also noted significant heterogeneity between included studies. The hazard ratio for development of NMSC was much higher in hospital-based studies compared with population-based studies, raising the possibility of both ascertainment bias (patients on thiopurines are more likely to be evaluated by a medical professional and thus be diagnosed with a medical condition) and surveillance bias (medical professionals aware of the association between thiopurines and NMSC may be more likely to examine for a skin condition and biopsy a suspicious lesion). Studies with shorter follow-up were also more likely to find a significant association between thiopurines and NMSC development for uncertain reasons. The authors concluded that while NMSC was associated with thiopurine use, the risk elevation was modest and should not preclude the use of these agents in the treatment of IBD.

Biologic Therapy and Skin Cancer

Whether biologic exposure is associated with an increased risk of skin cancer is not certain. As mentioned above, two of the larger studies to examine this issue in the IBD population had conflicting results. Long et al. found that the risk of melanoma was elevated in the IBD subpopulation receiving therapy with biologics with an odds ratio of 1.88 [61]. Similarly, a study that used the FDA Adverse Event Report System showed an increased risk of developing both melanoma and NMSC in IBD patients exposed to TNFα inhibitor compared to patients exposed to 5-ASA drugs [69]. On the other hand, a large systematic review and meta-analysis showed that the risk of melanoma was higher in the prebiologic era, implying that biologics may in some way be protective [62].

In contrast to the uncertainty in the IBD literature, in the rheumatologic literature, data suggests that TNFα inhibitor exposure is associated with development of both NMSC and melanoma. Indeed, one retrospective study found that, in the rheumatoid arthritis population (US prospective registry, $n = 13,001$), exposure to biologic therapy was associated with development of both melanoma (OR 2.3 [0.9–5.4 95% CI]) and NMSC (OR 1.5 [1.2–1.8 95% CI]) [70]. Infliximab had a stronger association than adalimumab, though numbers were small. A meta-analysis published in 2011 assessed the effect of anti-TNF exposure on development of all malignancies in the rheumatoid arthritis population examining only prospective studies and found no increased risk of malignancy, in general, with the exception of a clear association between anti-TNF and development of NMSC and a trend toward an association with melanoma [71]. Caution should be used in extrapolating these studies to the IBD population as the diseases themselves carry different risks of developing malignancy, irrespective of drug exposure.

The proposed biologic mechanism for the association between TNFα inhibition and melanoma involves cross-talk signaling between TNFα and IGF-1 (insulin-like growth factor). Overexposure to IGF-1 has been shown to enhance the proliferation of biologically early melanoma [72]. TNFα in vivo plays a role in downregulating IGF-1, and the introduction of TNFα binding proteins leads to an inability to engage in this role [73]. These findings suggest that patients exposed to TNFα inhibitors may have higher levels of circulating IGF-1 and thus enhanced risk of developing melanoma. Other authors point to a loss of immune surveillance, though experimental data for this theory is lacking.

In sum, while the totality of data in regards to the association between anti-TNFs and melanoma does not provide a clear picture, there is at least a signal toward an association. Given the morbidity associated with melanoma, caution should be exercised in choosing these agents in patients with a personal or family history of melanoma or who have multiple other risk factors. As always in treatment of IBD, a shared decision-making model of choosing a therapy, taking into account relative risks and benefits in the context of a patient's individual values, is considered best practice.

There is not enough data about methotrexate or newer biologics such as vedolizumab and ustekinumab to comment on their role in regards to development of skin cancer. This may highlight areas for future study.

IBD Subtype and Risk of Skin Cancer

Does IBD disease subtype play a role in the risk of developing skin cancer? There is a signal that Crohn's disease may be more strongly associated with melanoma than ulcerative colitis. A retrospective report using US population data showed that patients with Crohn's disease accounted for more of the excess risk of melanoma than patients with ulcerative colitis (CD IRR 1.45; 95% CI 1.13–1.85 vs UC IRR 1.13; 95% CI 0.89–1.42) [61]. A 2014 meta-analysis likewise showed an increased risk of melanoma in CD vs UC with a RR of 1.8 vs 1.2, respectively [62]. The explanation for increased risk in patients with CD is uncertain but may be speculated to be attributable either to different medication exposure (i.e., UC patients are more often managed with mesalamine monotherapy), pathophysiology of the disease itself, confounding risk factors (i.e., tobacco use in Crohn's disease), or healthcare utilization. More extensive IBD may put patients at an increased risk of developing melanoma [74]. This was demonstrated in both UC (pancolitis: cases 44.5% versus IBD controls without melanoma 28.1%; $p < 0.01$) and Crohn's disease (ileal and colonic disease: cases 57.9% versus controls 48.9%; $p = 0.02$). When compared to controls in the general population diagnosed with melanoma, IBD patients had similar survival.

Similarly, for NMSC, there appears to be a slightly increased risk of development of NMSC in Crohn's disease relative to ulcerative colitis. A 2010 meta-analysis found an SIR for development of squamous cell carcinoma for CD of 2.35 (95% CI 1.43–3.86), while the association for UC did not reach statistical significance (SIR 1.68; 95% CI 0.9–3.12) [59]. The University of Manitoba database similarly showed a slightly increased risk of NMSC in CD vs UC (1.38 vs 1.15, respectively) [58].

Risk of Second Skin Cancer in IBD Patients

It is well known that patients who have had one skin cancer have an increased risk of developing additional skin malignancies in the future [75–77]. It has been theorized that IBD patients may be prone to develop more skin cancers due to the inherent immune dysfunction in these patients compounded by the use of immuno-suppressive medications utilized in their treatment [62]. It would therefore follow that the risk of developing additional skin cancers in IBD patients would be higher than in skin cancer patients without IBD. There is however very little data published regarding the risk of a second skin cancer in patients with IBD, and what is available is controversial.

A number of studies have looked at the risk of incident cancers and recurrent cancers in IBD patients on antitumor necrosis factor alpha (anti-TNFα) medications and thiopurines, but the number of patients with skin cancer recurrences was limited, and the conclusions were difficult to interpret for skin cancer risk specifically [78, 79]. A study by a group at the University of Pennsylvania and the University of Alabama at Birmingham looked at the risk of developing a second non-melanoma skin cancer in patients with autoimmune disease treated with immunosuppressant or immunomodulatory medication. In this study, they looked at both IBD patients and patients with rheumatoid arthritis (RA). While anti-TNFα medications and metho-trexate were significantly associated with development of additional skin cancers in RA patients, the results were equivocal in IBD patients on thiopurines or anti-TNFα agents [80].

The authors of this chapter were unable to find studies to address the risk of developing an additional melanoma in IBD patients with a previous history of melanoma.

Does Risk Persist After Discontinuation of Immunosuppressive Agents?

An important consideration in clinical practice is whether discontinuation of a med-icine that has been associated with development of skin cancer will reduce the risk of a second skin cancer going forward. One case series with six patients in the transplant population showed decreased cutaneous carcinogenesis after discontinu-ation of immunosuppression [81]. In the CESAME cohort in France, a major find-ing was an increased hazard ratio for the development of NMSC in patients receiving current treatment with a thiopurine (5.9; 95% CI 2.13–16.4) and, notably, in patients with past treatment with a thiopurine (3.94; 95% CI 1.28–12.1) [66]. Another large study in the VA population had a conflicting result, demonstrating an elevated risk of developing NMSC while on thiopurines (HR 2.1, $p < 0.0001$) which went back to baseline after discontinuation (HR 0.7, $p = 0.07$) [67]. Given these conflicting results, it is difficult to draw definitive conclusions, but it seems prudent, in light of an increasing availability of therapeutic options for IBD beyond thiopurines, to strongly consider discontinuation of this modality of therapy in a patient who devel-ops an NMSC while on a thiopurine.

Management

Primary prevention is key in the management of skin cancers. Continued counseling by physicians regarding measures to reduce skin cancer risk in the IBD population is an important and simple intervention. These measures include strict photoprotection, avoiding tanning beds, stopping smoking, and regular self-skin checks. Photoprotection consists of three separate measures: avoiding outdoor sun during peak sun hours (from 10 am to 4 pm); wearing protective clothing including long sleeves, pants, wide brimmed hats, and sunglasses; and the regular application and reapplication of a broad-spectrum sunscreen between SPF 30 and 50 [42]. While the diagnosis and treatment of skin cancers often require the expertise of a dermatologist, all physicians can make a positive impact by counseling patients on the proper skin maintenance detailed above.

When a skin cancer is detected, the treatment depends on the type of skin cancer, including its size, location, and histopathologic features, within the context of the patient's preferences and medical comorbidities.

Non-melanoma Skin Cancer

Basal cell carcinoma can be successfully treated in a number of ways. Surgical options include electrodessication and curettage (ED&C), wide local excision (WLE) usually with a margin of 3–4 mm, or Mohs micrographic surgery. Other treatment options include cryotherapy, laser surgery, photodynamic therapy (PDT), topical chemotherapy, and radiation [77, 82]. Though rarely necessary, vismodegib, a targeted antagonist of the smoothened receptor within the hedgehog signaling pathway, is approved for use in patients who are not surgical candidates and for locally aggressive, surgically unresectable or metastatic disease [83].

Many of the above-described treatment modalities for BCC can also be used in the treatment of SCC. These include ED&C, WLE, Mohs surgery, cryotherapy, PDT, and topical chemotherapy. Radiation, chemotherapy, and biologics, like cetuximab, can be used as an adjunct to the surgical treatment of aggressive subtypes, recurrent disease, inoperable tumors or metastatic disease, and primarily in the case of nonsurgical candidates [77, 84].

Melanoma

The standard of care for the treatment of melanoma is wide local excision with margins determined by Breslow thickness. Margins range from 0.5 cm for in situ disease to 2 cm for deep lesions [85]. In cases of malignant melanoma in situ where the lesion is found on a cosmetically or functionally sensitive location, Mohs surgery or a staged excision (also known as slow Mohs) can be performed to ensure clearance while conserving as much normal skin as possible [86]. Sentinel lymph node biopsy is offered to aid staging if certain histopathologic features are considered unfavorable (advanced Breslow thickness and the presence of ulceration). Before 2011, options for metastatic or inoperable melanomas were severely limited. Since that time, targeted therapy and immunotherapies including immune checkpoint inhibitors and oncolytic viral therapy have been approved for use in these patients with good success [85].

Immunosuppressive Medications in Skin Cancer Patients with IBD

Currently, there are no published guidelines that recommend an altered approach to the management of skin cancers in patients carrying a diagnosis of IBD. That being said, the authors feel that patients' concurrent medical problems and medications should be taken into account when directing therapy. IBD patients, for example, are often considered immunocompromised due to their medications. Immunocompromised patients are typically monitored more closely and treated more aggressively as it is understood that their innate cancer surveillance is hampered [22, 42, 86]. The initiation or continuation of immunosuppressive agents should therefore be considered carefully in IBD patients who develop skin cancers.

Swoger and Regueiro recently published a review article specifically aimed at decisions regarding immunomodulatory and biologic therapies in IBD patients in whom an infection or malignancy had developed [87]. The authors acknowledge the known association of thiopurines with increased risk of non-melanoma skin cancer. However, stopping these therapies has not been definitively shown to improve current tumors or future risk of developing new tumors [66]. As a result, a measured approach to these patients was suggested by the authors. In patients with a previous diagnosis of NMSC, the initiation of azathioprine or mercaptopurine (AZA/6MP) should take into account the severity of the prior cancer. For patients who develop NMSC during therapy, the recommendation is to continue AZA/6MP as long as the lesions are not high risk in nature and can be easily addressed with local treatment. If this is not the case, the use of AZA/6MP should be reconsidered. As TNFα inhibitors and methotrexate are less strongly associated with the development of NMSC, the recommendation is to start these medications in patients with NMSC history but with close dermatologic follow-up. Melanoma, however, requires a stricter approach. Swoger and Reguerio recommend avoiding the initiation of immunosuppressive agents for 2 years following the successful treatment of a melanoma and stopping any immunosuppressive therapy on the diagnosis of a new melanoma. They also recommend that immunosuppressive medications should not be used in patients with metastatic disease. Limiting other potential iatrogenic risks should also be considered. A skin cancer patient with concurrent IBD and psoriasis, for example, would not be the best candidate for phototherapy.

Screening Recommendations for IBD Patients

There is mixed evidence regarding the usefulness of annual full skin checks conducted by a physician in the general adult population. The US Preventative Services Task Force (USPSTF) reviewed the literature in 2001 and again in 2009 and found insufficient evidence to make a recommendation regarding regular full skin exams for the early detection of skin cancers [88].

However, as discussed already, patients with inflammatory bowel disease are at an increased risk for the development of melanoma and non-melanoma skin cancers both inherently and due to commonly utilized immunomodulatory and immunosuppressive medications. Thus, recommendations regarding the general US adult population are too broad to apply to this special group. Many in clinical practice recommend that patients with IBD perform regular self-skin exams and have yearly physician-conducted full skin exams [79, 87, 89–91]. The authors of this chapter are in agreement with this, but consideration should be given that the yearly full skin exam be conducted by a dermatologist. Studies have shown that patients who perform self-skin checks and who have regular checks by dermatologists have thinner melanomas at diagnosis when compared to patients who did not take these measures [92, 93]. The presumption is that the melanomas are detected at an earlier stage. Certainly IBD patients with multiple risk factors for skin cancer such as chronic sun exposure, family history of skin cancer, multiple nevi, or long history of immune suppression would likely benefit from more frequent skin checks by a dermatologist. Okafor et al. published a mathematical model that supported yearly total body skin exams by a physician as the most cost-effective option for the detection and treatment of non-melanoma skin cancers in IBD patients [94]. Once a skin cancer is detected, the frequency of full body skin exams is carried out by a dermatologist as per the national guidelines.

All dermatologic evaluations should include careful observation and palpation of scars from prior skin cancer surgeries in order to detect possible recurrence. Additionally, every patient with a history of melanoma should have a lymph node exam as part of their regular dermatology visit. Self-skin checks performed by the patient should continue on a monthly basis following a skin cancer diagnosis as an adjunct to physician visits [93]. Patients can be instructed on how to use mirrors to examine areas that are difficult to visualize such as the back. Alternatively, a family member or close friend could serve as an additional screener, comparing the patient's current appearance to a previous baseline photo. Patients should be instructed regarding what constitutes a concerning lesion that requires prompt review by a dermatologist. Any lesions that persistently hurt, itch, bleed, do not heal, continue to grow, or moles that meet the ABCDE criteria (asymmetry, irregular borders, multiple colors, diameter >6 mm, evolving), should be evaluated by a

Table 3.2 Summary of recommendations for IBD patients

Recommendation	Notes
Counsel patients on primary prevention	Includes photoprotective behaviors, avoiding smoking, avoiding tanning beds
Counsel patients on photoprotection strategies	Seek shade when possible, avoid sun exposure during peak hours, wear protective clothing, use broad-spectrum sunscreen (SPF 30–50)
Perform self-skin checks	Ideally monthly
Annual full skin exam by physician	Applies to all patients with IBD given increased risk of melanoma. Consideration given to being performed by dermatologist (especially in high-risk individuals, i.e., fair skin, greater than 50, on thiopurine)
Consider modifying therapy in patient diagnosed with NMSC on a thiopurine, especially if aggressive or multiple	Review with patient's dermatologist. Data conflicting about what happens to the risk of new NMSC after thiopurine discontinuation
Consider stopping immunosuppression if diagnosed with melanoma, especially TNFα inhibitors. Consider avoiding starting TNFα inhibitor in patient with personal history of melanoma	Some data suggest increased risk of melanoma development in patients treated with TNFα inhibitors. Little data about risk after discontinuation

dermatologist immediately [95, 96]. Patients should be instructed to adopt a low threshold for seeing a dermatologist should they notice any of these features. Table 3.2 summarizes recommendations for best practices in regards to skin cancer risk and management for IBD patients.

Conclusion

The most commonly encountered skin cancers are BCC, cutaneous SCC, and melanoma. BCC and SCC are frequently encountered but thankfully have low morbidity if they are caught early and are of low-risk subtypes. They can however be locally invasive and cause significant morbidity depending on their location, size, and histologic subtypes and have the potential to result in large disfiguring surgical defects. Mortality, however, is overall very low. Melanoma, on the other hand, especially when at an advanced stage, carries a grim prognosis. IBD is associated with the development of both melanoma and NMSC, with IBD itself appearing to be a risk factor for melanoma while the excess risk of NMSC is likely mostly attributable to exposure to thiopurines. TNFα inhibitors may also be associated with the development of melanoma, though data is conflicting. Despite these associations, IBD patients receive lower levels of dermatologic care and less skin cancer screening than recommended [97].

IBD practitioners should be aware of these associations and be alert when gathering patient history and planning treatment strategies for their patients. Given the availability of other steroid-sparing options for IBD, consideration can be given to avoiding thiopurines in patients with a personal history of NMSC or a strong family history of the same or multiple other risk factors. Additionally, all IBD patients should be apprised of recommendations for primary prevention of skin cancer, including photoprotective behaviors, monthly self-skin exams, and undergoing an annual total body skin exam with a dermatologist. The latter behavior has been associated with thinner melanomas at diagnosis, presumably from earlier diagnosis.

Treatment of skin cancer, once diagnosed, is often coordinated by dermatology. Thin melanomas and NMSC are primarily handled by dermatology. More advanced melanomas and aggressive SCC often require a multidisciplinary approach, potentially including surgery, oncology, and radiation oncology. Management of medications for treatment of IBD after a diagnosis of skin cancer requires a multidisciplinary understanding of the disease process, typically involving discussion between the dermatologist and the gastroenterologist, and takes into account relative risks and benefits of different approaches in the context of the patient's values.

Disclosures No relevant disclosures.

References

1. Rogers HW, Weinstock MA, Feldman SR, Coldiron BM. Incidence estimate of nonmelanoma skin cancer (keratinocyte carcinomas) in the US population, 2012. JAMA Dermatol. 2015;151:1081–6.
2. Housman TS, et al. Skin cancer is among the most costly of all cancers to treat for the Medicare population. J Am Acad Dermatol. 2003;48:425–9.
3. Euvrard S, Kanitakis J, Claudy A. Skin cancers after organ transplantation. N Engl J Med. 2003;348:1681–91.
4. Fortina AB, et al. Immunosuppressive level and other risk factors for basal cell carcinoma and squamous cell carcinoma in heart transplant recipients. Arch Dermatol. 2004;140:1079–85.
5. Byun J, et al. Clinical outcomes of primary intracranial malignant melanoma and metastatic intracranial malignant melanoma. Clin Neurol Neurosurg. 2018;164:32–8.
6. Helgadottir H, Drakensjo IRT, Girnita A. Personalized medicine in malignant melanoma: towards patient tailored treatment. Front Oncol. 2018;8:1–15.
7. Cameron MC, et al. Basal cell carcinoma: part 1. J Am Acad Dermatol. 2018; https://doi.org/10.1016/j.jaad.2018.03.060.
8. Sexton M, Jones DB, Maloney ME. Histologic pattern analysis of basal cell carcinoma: study of a series of 1039 consecutive neoplasms. J Am Acad Dermatol. 1990;23:1118–26.
9. Zanetti R, et al. Comparison of risk patterns in carcinoma and melanoma of the skin in men: a multi-centre case–case–control study. Br J Cancer. 2006;94:743–51.
10. Szewczyk M, et al. Basal cell carcinoma in farmers: an occupation group at high risk. Int Arch Occup Environ Health. 2016;89:497–501.
11. Kaskel P, et al. Ultraviolet exposure and risk of melanoma and basal cell carcinoma in Ulm and Dresden, Germany. J Eur Acad Dermatol Venereol. 2018;29:134–42.
12. Lomas A, Leonardi-Bee J, Bath-Hextall F. A systematic review of worldwide incidence of nonmelanoma skin cancer. Br J Dermatol. 2018;166:1069–80.
13. Zalaudek I, et al. Dermoscopy of Bowen's disease. Br J Dermatol. 2004;150:1112–6.

14. Edwards MJ, Hirsch RM, Broadwater JR, Netscher DT, Ames FC. Squamous cell carcinoma arising in previously burned or irradiated skin. Arch Surg. 1989;124:115–7.
15. Brantsch KD, et al. Analysis of risk factors determining prognosis of cutaneous squamous-cell carcinoma: a prospective study. Lancet Oncol. 2008;9:713–20.
16. Breuninger H, Schaumburg-Lever G, Holzschuh J, Horny H-P. Desmoplastic squamous cell carcinoma of skin and vermilion surface. Cancer. 1997;79:915–9.
17. Azorín D, López-Ríos F, Ballestín C, Barrientos N, Rodríguez-Peralto JL. Primary cutaneous adenosquamous carcinoma: a case report and review of the literature. J Cutan Pathol. 2001;28:542–5.
18. Almahroos M, Kurban AK. Ultraviolet carcinogenesis in nonmelanoma skin cancer. Part I: incidence rates in relation to geographic locations and in migrant populations. Skinmed. 2004;3:29–35.
19. Chen GJ, et al. Clinical diagnosis of actinic keratosis identifies an elderly population at high risk of developing skin cancer. Dermatol Surg. 2005;31:43–7.
20. zur Hausen H. Papillomaviruses in the causation of human cancers – a brief historical account. Virology. 2009;384:260–5.
21. Xiang F, Lucas R, Hales S, Neale R. Incidence of nonmelanoma skin cancer in relation to ambient UV radiation in white populations, 1978–2012: empirical relationships. JAMA Dermatol. 2014;150:1063–71.
22. Rowe DE, Carroll RJ, Day CL. Prognostic factors for local recurrence, metastasis and survival rates in squamous cell carcinoma of the skin, ear, and lip. J Am Acad Dermatol. 1992;26:976–90.
23. Yuspa SH. Cutaneous chemical carcinogenesis. J Am Acad Dermatol. 1986;15:1031–44.
24. Jensen P, et al. Skin cancer in kidney and heart transplant recipients and different long-term immunosuppressive therapy regimens. J Am Acad Dermatol. 1999;40:177–86.
25. Hartevelt MM, Bavinck JN, Vandenbroucke JP. Incidence of skin cancer after renal transplantation in the Netherlands. Transplantation. 1990;49:506–9.
26. Lindelöf B, Sigurgeirsson B, Gäbel H, Stern RS. Incidence of skin cancer in 5356 patients following organ transplantation. Br J Dermatol. 2018;143:513–9.
27. Velez NF, et al. Association of advanced leukemic stage and skin cancer tumor stage with poor skin cancer outcomes in patients with chronic lymphocytic leukemia. JAMA Dermatol. 2014;150:280–7.
28. Mehrany K, Weenig RH, Pittelkow MR, Roenigk RK, Otley CC. High recurrence rates of squamous cell carcinoma after Mohs' surgery in patients with chronic lymphocytic leukemia. Dermatol Surg. 2018;31:38–42.
29. Weinberg AS, Ogle CA, Shim EK. Metastatic cutaneous squamous cell carcinoma: an update. Dermatol Surg. 2018;33:885–99.
30. Staples M, Marks R, Giles G. Trends in the incidence of non-melanocytic skin cancer (NMSC) treated in Australia 1985–1995: are primary prevention programs starting to have an effect? Int J Cancer. 1998;78:144–8.
31. Nestor MS, Zarraga MB. The incidence of nonmelanoma skin cancers and actinic keratoses in South Florida. J Clin Aesthet Dermatol. 2012;5:20–4.
32. Mudigonda T, Pearce DJ, Yentzer BA. The economic impact of non-melanoma skin cancer: a review. J Natl Compr Cancer Netw. 2010;8:888–97.
33. Weinstock MA. Nonmelanoma skin cancer mortality in the United States, 1969 through 1988. Arch Dermatol. 1993;129:1286–90.
34. Rigel DS, Friedman RJ, Kopf AW. Lifetime risk for development of skin cancer in the U.S. population: current estimate is now 1 in 5. J Am Acad Dermatol. 1996;35:1012–3.
35. Rubin AI, Chen EH, Ratner D. Basal-cell carcinoma. N Engl J Med. 2005;353:2262–9.
36. Lewis KG, Weinstock MA. Nonmelanoma skin Cancer mortality (1988–2000): the Rhode Island follow-back study. Arch Dermatol. 2004;140:837–42.
37. Karia PS, Han J, Schmults CD. Cutaneous squamous cell carcinoma: estimated incidence of disease, nodal metastasis, and deaths from disease in the United States, 2012. J Am Acad Dermatol. 2013;68:957–66.

38. Guy GP, Machlin SR, Ekwueme DU, Yabroff KR. Prevalence and costs of skin cancer treatment in the U.S., 2002–2006 and 2007–2011. Am J Prev Med. 2015;48:183–7.
39. Pizzichetta MA, et al. Dermoscopic diagnosis of amelanotic/hypomelanotic melanoma. Br J Dermatol. 2018;177:538–40.
40. Melanoma of the skin – cancer stat facts; 2018. https://seer.cancer.gov/statfacts/html/melan.html. Accessed 29 July 2018.
41. Garbe C, Leiter U. Melanoma epidemiology and trends. Clin Dermatol. 2009;27:3–9.
42. Key statistics for melanoma skin cancer; 2018. https://www.cancer.org/cancer/melanoma-skin-cancer/about/key-statistics.html. Accessed 29 July 2018.
43. Berwick M, et al. Melanoma epidemiology and prevention. Can Treat Res. 2016;167:17–49.
44. Gandini S, et al. Meta-analysis of risk factors for cutaneous melanoma: II. Sun exposure. Eur J Cancer. 2005;41:45–60.
45. Lazovich D, et al. Association between indoor tanning and melanoma in younger men and women. JAMA Dermatol. 2016;152:268–75.
46. Gandini S, et al. Meta-analysis of risk factors for cutaneous melanoma: I. Common and atypical naevi. Eur J Cancer. 2005;41:28–44.
47. Ransohoff KJ, et al. Familial skin cancer syndromes: increased melanoma risk. J Am Acad Dermatol. 2016;74:423–34.
48. Ariyan S, Kluger H. eds. The melanoma handbook. New York: Springer; 2017.
49. Bolognia JL, Jorizzo JL, Schaffer JV. *Dermatology*. Philadelphia: Elsevier, Saunders; 2012.
50. Erdei E, Torres SM. A new understanding in the epidemiology of melanoma. Expert Rev Anticancer Ther. 2010;10:1811–23.
51. Lasithiotakis K, et al. Age and gender are significant independent predictors of survival in primary cutaneous melanoma. Cancer. 2008;112:1795–804.
52. Buettner PG, Leiter U, Eigentler TK, Garbe C. Development of prognostic factors and survival in cutaneous melanoma over 25 years. Cancer. 2018;103:616–24.
53. Linos E, Swetter SM, Cockburn MG, Colditz GA, Clarke CA. Increasing burden of melanoma in the United States. J Invest Dermatol. 2009;129:1666–74.
54. Rouhani P, Hu S, Kirsner RS. Melanoma in Hispanic and black Americans, melanoma in Hispanic and black Americans. Cancer Control. 2008;15:248–53.
55. Mora RG, Perniciaro C. Cancer of the skin in blacks. I. A review of 163 black patients with cutaneous squamous cell carcinoma. J Am Acad Dermatol. 1981;5:535–43.
56. Ekbom A, Helmick C, Zack M, Adami HO. Extracolonic malignancies in inflammatory bowel disease. Cancer. 1991;67:2015–9.
57. Jess T, Winther KV, Munkholm P, Langholz E, Binder V. Intestinal and extra-intestinal cancer in Crohn's disease: follow-up of a population-based cohort in Copenhagen County, Denmark. Aliment Pharmacol Ther. 2004;19:287–93.
58. Bernstein CN, Blanchard JF, Kliewer E, Wajda A. Cancer risk in patients with inflammatory bowel disease: a population-based study. Cancer. 2001;91:854–62.
59. Pedersen N, et al. Risk of extra-intestinal cancer in inflammatory bowel disease: meta-analysis of population-based cohort studies. Am J Gastroenterol. 2010;105:1480–7.
60. Kappelman MD, et al. Risk of cancer in patients with inflammatory bowel diseases: a nationwide population-based cohort study with 30 years of follow-up evaluation. Clin Gastroenterol Hepatol. 2014;12:265–73.e1.
61. Long MD, et al. Risk of melanoma and nonmelanoma skin Cancer among patients with inflammatory bowel disease. Gastroenterology. 2012;143:390–399.e1.
62. Singh S, et al. Inflammatory bowel disease is associated with an increased risk of melanoma: a systematic review and meta-analysis. Clin Gastroenterol Hepatol. 2014;12:210–8.
63. O'Donovan P, et al. Azathioprine and UVA light generate mutagenic oxidative DNA damage. Science. 2005;309:1871–4.
64. Perrett CM, et al. Azathioprine treatment photosensitizes human skin to ultraviolet a radiation. Br J Dermatol. 2008;159:198–204.
65. Harwood C, et al. PTCH mutations in basal cell carcinomas from azathioprine-treated organ transplant recipients. Br J Cancer. 2008;99:1276–84.

66. Peyrin-Biroulet L, et al. Increased risk for nonmelanoma skin cancers in patients who receive thiopurines for inflammatory bowel disease. Gastroenterology. 2011;141:1621–28.e1–5.
67. Abbas AM, Almukhtar RM, Loftus EV, Lichtenstein GR, Khan N. Risk of melanoma and non-melanoma skin cancer in ulcerative colitis patients treated with thiopurines: a nationwide retrospective cohort. Am J Gastroenterol. 2014;109:1781–93.
68. Ariyaratnam J, Subramanian V. Association between thiopurine use and nonmelanoma skin cancers in patients with inflammatory bowel disease: a meta-analysis. Am J Gastroenterol. 2014;109:163–9.
69. McKenna MR, Stobaugh DJ, Deepak P. Melanoma and non-melanoma skin cancer in inflammatory bowel disease patients following tumor necrosis factor-α inhibitor monotherapy and in combination with thiopurines: analysis of the food and drug administration adverse event reporting system. J Gastrointest Liver Dis. 2014;23:267.
70. Wolfe F, Michaud K. Biologic treatment of rheumatoid arthritis and the risk of malignancy: analyses from a large US observational study. Arthritis Rheum. 2007;56:2886–95.
71. Mariette X, et al. Malignancies associated with tumour necrosis factor inhibitors in registries and prospective observational studies: a systematic review and meta-analysis. Ann Rheum Dis. 2011;70:1895–904.
72. Satyamoorthy K, Li G, Vaidya B, Patel D, Herlyn M. Insulin-like growth factor-1 induces survival and growth of biologically early melanoma cells through both the mitogen-activated protein kinase and beta-catenin pathways. Cancer Res. 2001;61:7318–24.
73. Frost RA, Nystrom GJ, Lang CH. Tumor necrosis factor-α decreases insulin-like growth factor-I messenger ribonucleic acid expression in C2C12 myoblasts via a Jun N-terminal kinase pathway. Endocrinology. 2003;144:1770–9.
74. Nissen LHC, et al. Risk factors and clinical outcomes in patients with IBD with melanoma. Inflamm Bowel Dis. 2017;23:2018–26.
75. Rees JR, et al. Non melanoma skin cancer and subsequent cancer risk. PLoS One. 2014;9:e99674.
76. Hallaji Z, Rahimi H, Mirshams-Shahshahani M. Comparison of risk factors of single basal cell carcinoma with multiple basal cell carcinomas. Indian J Dermatol. 2011;56:398–402.
77. Preston DS, Stern RS. Nonmelanoma cancers of the skin. N Engl J Med. 1992;327:1649–62.
78. Poullenot F, et al. Risk of incident cancer in inflammatory bowel disease patients starting anti-TNF therapy while having recent malignancy. Inflamm Bowel Dis. 2016;22:1362–9.
79. Beaugerie L, et al. Risk of new or recurrent cancer under immunosuppressive therapy in patients with IBD and previous cancer. Gut. 2014;63:1416–23.
80. Scott FI, et al. Risk of nonmelanoma skin cancer associated with the use of immunosuppressant and biologic agents in patients with a history of autoimmune disease and nonmelanoma skin cancer. JAMA Dermatol. 2016;152:164–72.
81. Otley CC, Coldiron BM, Stasko T, Goldman GD. Decreased skin cancer after cessation of therapy with transplant-associated immunosuppressants. Arch Dermatol. 2001;137:459–63.
82. Cameron MC, et al. Basal cell carcinoma, part II: contemporary approaches to diagnosis, treatment, and prevention. J Am Acad Dermatol. 2018; https://doi.org/10.1016/j.jaad.2018.02.083.
83. Basset-Séguin N, et al. Vismodegib in patients with advanced basal cell carcinoma: primary analysis of STEVIE, an international, open-label trial. Eur J Cancer. 2017;86:334–48.
84. Scarpati GDV, Perri F, Pisconti S. Concomitant cetuximab and radiation therapy: a possible promising strategy for locally advanced inoperable non-melanoma skin carcinomas. Mol Clin Oncol. 2016;4:467–71.
85. NCCN – Evidence-based cancer guidelines, oncology drug compendium, oncology continuing medical education. NCCN guidelines melanoma; 2018.
86. Connolly AHTFSM, et al. AAD/ACMS/ASDSA/ASMS 2012 appropriate use criteria for Mohs micrographic surgery: a report of the American Academy of Dermatology, American College of Mohs Surgery, American Society for Dermatologic Surgery Association, and the American Society for Mohs Su. Dermatol Surg. 2012;38:1582–603.

87. Swoger JM, Regueiro M. Stopping, continuing, or restarting immunomodulators and biologics when an infection or malignancy develops. Inflamm Bowel Dis. 2014;20:926–35.
88. Grossman DC, et al. Behavioral counseling to prevent skin cancer. JAMA. 2018;319:1134.
89. Kasiske BL, et al. Recommendations for the outpatient surveillance of renal transplant recipients. J Am Soc Nephrol. 2000;11:S1–S86.
90. Abegunde AT, Muhammad BH, Ali T. Preventive health measures in inflammatory bowel disease. World J Gastroenterol. 2016;22:7625–44.
91. Farraye FA, Melmed GY, Lichtenstein GR, Kane SV. ACG clinical guideline: preventive care in inflammatory bowel disease. Am J Gastroenterol. 2017;112:241.
92. Aitken JF, Elwood M, Baade PD, Youl P, English D. Clinical whole-body skin examination reduces the incidence of thick melanomas. Int J Cancer. 2009;126:450–8.
93. Swetter SM, Pollitt RA, Johnson TM, Brooks DR, Geller AC. Behavioral determinants of successful early melanoma detection. Cancer. 2011;118:3725–34.
94. Okafor PN, et al. Cost-effectiveness of nonmelanoma skin cancer screening in Crohn's disease patients. Inflamm Bowel Dis. 2013;19:2787–95.
95. Marghoob AA, Scope A. The complexity of diagnosing melanoma. J Invest Dermatol. 2009;129:11–3.
96. Condon C. Learning your ABCDEs of melanoma. Irish Med Times. 2016;50:33.
97. Anderson A, et al. Low rates of dermatologic care and skin cancer screening among inflammatory bowel disease patients. Dig Dis Sci. 2018:1–11; https://doi.org/10.1007/s10620-018-5056-x.

Chapter 4
Female-Specific Cancer Risks and Screening in Inflammatory Bowel Disease

Kara De Felice and Sunanda Kane

Cervical Cancer

Cervical cancer is the fourth most frequent cancer in women worldwide. There were an estimated 527,600 new cervical cancer cases and 265,700 cervical cancer deaths worldwide in 2012. Cervical cancer is caused by persistent infection with oncogenic human papilloma virus (HPV). Smoking and a compromised immune system increase the risk for cancer development [1].

The data regarding an increased risk of cervical dysplasia and cancer from simply having a diagnosis of IBD are conflicting, but there is a consistent trend for the increased risk associated with the use of immunosuppressants.

A nationwide cohort study from Denmark matched 26,000 women with IBD with the general population (N = 1,508,000). Women with UC had an increased risk of low-grade (IRR 1.15, 1.00–1.32) and high-grade lesions (IRR 1.12, 1.01–1.25) compared to healthy controls. Women with CD had increased risk of low-grade lesions (1.26, 1.07–1.48), high-grade lesions (IRR 1.28, 1.13–1.45), and cervical cancer (IRR 1.53, 1.04–2.27) [2]. This increased risk was not found in a large Canadian population-based study [3].

A meta-analysis of eight studies found sufficient evidence to suggest an increased risk of cervical high-grade dysplasia and cancer in patients with IBD on immunosuppressive medications with an adjusted odds ratio of 1.34 (1.23–1.46) [4]. However, the analysis did not specify medication type, dose, or duration.

Thiopurine exposure appears to carry a higher risk of cervical dysplasia and cancer compared to anti-TNF and vedolizumab exposure [2, 5–8]. No cervical

K. De Felice (✉)
Louisiana State University Health Science Center, New Orleans, LA, USA
e-mail: kdefel@lsuhsc.edu

S. Kane
Mayo Clinic, Rochester, MN, USA
e-mail: kane.sunanda@mayo.edu

© Springer Nature Switzerland AG 2019
J. D. Feuerstein, A. S. Cheifetz (eds.), *Cancer Screening in Inflammatory Bowel Disease*, https://doi.org/10.1007/978-3-030-15301-4_4

cancer cases have been reported with ustekinumab and tofacitinib in IBD patients to date, but the experience with these agents is limited [9, 10].

Cervical Cancer Screening

Women with IBD should be screened according to guidelines directed at those with a history of immunosuppression. The Centers for Disease Control American Cancer Society and American Congress of Obstetricians and Gynecologists support annual cervical cancer screening intervals for patients on chronic immunosuppression [11].

Preventative care for HPV vaccination should be offered to every female with IBD, ages 9–45, regardless of their medical therapy.

Vulvovaginal Cancer

Vulvovaginal cancer is rare and accounts for <1% of all female cancers; however, the incidence rates are rising. Risk factors are HPV infection, smoking, cervical cancer, and lichen sclerosis [12].

The risk of vulvovaginal cancer in IBD patients and the influence of immunosuppressive medications are largely unknown as this cancer is rare and limited data available.

In a retrospective single-center study, more cases of vulvovaginal cancer were found in CD patients but not in UC patients [13]. Another retrospective study reports one case of vulvar cancer in a cohort of 1248 UC patients [14].

Vulvovaginal Cancer Screening

There are no specific guidelines for vulvovaginal screening; however, annual speculum and bimanual pelvic exams as part of cervical cancer screening are indicated for IBD patients who are immunosuppressed. HPV is a risk factor for vulvovaginal cancer, and HPV vaccines should be offered to IBD women (ages 9–45) for prevention [11].

Ovarian Cancer

Ovarian cancer incidence rates are rising worldwide. There were an estimated 238,700 new ovarian cancer cases and 151,900 ovarian cancer deaths worldwide in 2012. Risk factors include smoking, early menarche, late menopause, nulliparity, polycystic ovarian syndrome, endometriosis, and genetic susceptibility [1].

Literature on ovarian cancer in IBD patients is again limited. In general, the risk of ovarian cancer in IBD patients is similar to the general population. There may be a small increase in risk with thiopurines; however the data is scarce. Anti-TNF and vedolizumab have not been associated with an increased risk.

Large population-based studies from Sweden, Denmark, and Spain found a similar risk of ovarian cancer in IBD patients compared to the general population [15–17]. Similarly, a meta-analysis of 17,000 IBD patients did not find an increased risk of ovarian cancer [18].

Anti-TNF exposure has not been associated with an increased risk of ovarian cancer in a large nationwide register-based cohort study of 56,146 IBD patients [19]. In a systemic review and meta-analysis of six randomized controlled trials and recent publication on the long-term safety data on vedolizumab, there has been no reports on ovarian cancer [20, 21]. No cases of ovarian cancer were reported in the OCTAVE and UNITI trials for tofacitinib and ustekinumab [9, 10].

In a small study, two ovarian cancers were reported in the thiopurine-exposed group compared to those without thiopurine exposure [22]. A large Danish cohort also reported a higher occurrence of female genital organ cancers in thiopurine-exposed patients compared to the unexposed patients [23].

Ovarian Cancer Screening

Regular screening for ovarian cancer in IBD patients with or without immunosuppressive drugs is not recommended.

Endometrial Cancer

Worldwide, in 2012, 527,600 women were diagnosed with endometrial cancer. The mortality rate was 1.7–2.4 per 100,000 women. Risk factors include age above 55, estrogen exposure, obesity, early menarche, late menopause, nulliparity, tamoxifen therapy, and genetic susceptibility [1].

Literature on endometrial cancer in IBD patients is scarce. In general, the risk of endometrial cancer in IBD patients is similar to the general population regardless of immunosuppressive agents.

Earlier studies reported a higher risk of endometrial cancer in UC patients; however, these findings have not been confirmed in more recent studies [14, 16, 18, 24]. A meta-analysis of extraintestinal malignancies in IBD patients reports an incidental risk of endometrial cancer in IBD (SIR 0.9, 95% CI 0.49–1.75), CD (SIR 0.84, 95% CI 0.36–1.96), and UC (SIR 1.12, 95% CI 0.54–2.32) patients [18].

Several studies have not found an increased risk of endometrial cancer with anti-TNF agents [24–26]. There have been no reports of thiopurine-, vedolizumab-, ustekinumab-, and tofacitinib-associated risks of endometrial cancer [7, 9, 10, 21].

Endometrial Cancer Screening

Regular screening for endometrial cancer in IBD patients with or without immuno-suppressive drugs is not recommended.

Breast Cancer

Breast cancer is the most frequently diagnosed cancer and the leading cause of cancer death among females worldwide, with an estimated 1.7 million cases and 521,900 deaths in 2012. Risk factors include early menarche, late menopause, oral contraceptive use, hormone replacement therapy, nulliparity or late first birth, obesity, genetic susceptibility, family history, physical inactivity, and alcohol [1].

The risk of breast cancer in IBD patients seems to be similar to the general population, and it may be decreased for CD. There are no studies primarily assessing the risk and risk factors of breast cancer in IBD patients, and most data are derived from population-based cohort studies.

A meta-analysis of eight population-based cohort studies found no difference in the occurrence of breast cancer in both UC and CD compared to the general population [18]. A Spanish cohort study showed a declined risk of breast cancer in IBD patients compared to the general population (RR 0.63, 95% CI 0.32–0.89) [17]. The TREAT cohort registry, a long-term safety registry of patients treated with infliximab versus other medications, found a SIR of 0.28 (95% CI 0.08–0.72) [16]. Similarly, the Dutch Inflammatory Bowel Disease South Limburg cohort reported a SIR of 0.11 (95% CI 0.00–0.64) and a Swedish population-based cohort a SIR of 0.85 (95% CI 0.75–0.97) [24, 27].

Anti-TNF agents and vedolizumab have not been associated with breast cancer development [20, 28]. Thiopurine exposure has been associated with an increase in solid malignancy in general; however, there has been no direct association between thiopurines and breast cancer development [22, 23, 29].

A large Danish cohort study (56,146 IBD patients) found no difference in the incidence of breast cancer in anti-TNF-exposed patients compared to nonexposed patients [19]. The TREAT registry CD cohort found a decrease in the occurrence of breast cancer in the infliximab-exposed (SIR 0.5, 95% CI 0.24–0.92) and unexposed (SIR 0.32, 95% CI 0.12–0.70) IBD patients compared to the general population [24]. A meta-analysis of 22 randomized controlled trials found no difference in breast cancer between anti-TNF therapy (one case) and placebo (three cases) [28].

There is limited information with the use of vedolizumab. Two out of 2830 IBD patients treated with vedolizumab were found to have breast cancer. Both patients had previously been exposed to other immunosuppressive medications [20].

Long-term data for tofacitinib and ustekinumab are lacking; however, there were no reports of breast cancer in the OCTAVE and UNITI trials [9, 10].

There has been no clear association between thiopurine use and breast cancer development. Both a Danish and British cohort did not find an increased risk of breast cancer in those exposed to thiopurines [22, 23, 29].

Breast Cancer Screening

Earlier and more frequent breast cancer screening is not recommended for IBD patients at this time.

A population-based study found that there were no significant differences in the use of mammograms in women with or without IBD. However, only 47% of women with IBD had mammograms regularly [5].

The US Preventative Services Task Force recommends biennial screening mammography for women aged 50–74 years. This recommendation applies to asymptomatic women with no risk factors for breast cancer (preexisting high-risk breast lesion, history of breast cancer, history of chest radiation, genetic markers for breast cancer such as BRCA1/BRAC2). The decision to start screening mammography in women prior to age 50 years should be an individualized based on their risk factors [30].

References

1. Torre LA, Bray F, Siegel RL, Ferlay J, Lortet-Tieulent J, Jemal A. Global cancer statistics, 2012. CA Cancer J Clin. 2015;65(2):87–108.
2. Rungoe C, Simonsen J, Riis L, Frisch M, Langholz E, Jess T. Inflammatory bowel disease and cervical neoplasia: a population-based nationwide cohort study. Clin Gastroenterol Hepatol. 2015;13(4):693–700.e1.
3. Singh H, Demers AA, Nugent Z, Mahmud SM, Kliewer EV, Bernstein CN. Risk of cervical abnormalities in women with inflammatory bowel disease: a population-based nested case-control study. Gastroenterology. 2009;136(2):451–8.
4. Allegretti JR, Barnes EL, Cameron A. Are patients with inflammatory bowel disease on chronic immunosuppressive therapy at increased risk of cervical high-grade dysplasia/cancer? A meta-analysis. Inflamm Bowel Dis. 2015;21(5):1089–97.
5. Singh H, Nugent Z, Demers AA, Bernstein CN. Screening for cervical and breast cancer among women with inflammatory bowel disease: a population-based study. Inflamm Bowel Dis. 2011;17(8):1741–50.
6. Dugue PA, Rebolj M, Hallas J, Garred P, Lynge E. Risk of cervical cancer in women with auto-immune diseases, in relation with their use of immunosuppressants and screening: population-based cohort study. Int J Cancer. 2015;136(6):E711–9.
7. Luthra P, Peyrin-Biroulet L, Ford AC. Systematic review and meta-analysis: opportunistic infections and malignancies during treatment with anti-integrin antibodies in inflammatory bowel disease. Aliment Pharmacol Ther. 2015;41(12):1227–36.
8. Osterman MT, Sandborn WJ, Colombel JF, Robinson AM, Lau W, Huang B, et al. Increased risk of malignancy with adalimumab combination therapy, compared with monotherapy, for Crohn's disease. Gastroenterology. 2014;146(4):941–9.
9. Feagan BG, Sandborn WJ, Gasink C, Jacobstein D, Lang Y, Friedman JR, et al. Ustekinumab as induction and maintenance therapy for Crohn's disease. N Engl J Med. 2016;375(20):1946–60.

10. Sandborn WJ, Su C, Sands BE, D'Haens GR, Vermeire S, Schreiber S, et al. Tofacitinib as induction and maintenance therapy for ulcerative colitis. N Engl J Med. 2017;376(18):1723–36.
11. Farraye FA, Melmed GY, Lichtenstein GR, Kane SV. ACG clinical guideline: preventive care in inflammatory bowel disease. Am J Gastroenterol. 2017;112(2):241–58.
12. Dittmer C, Katalinic A, Mundhenke C, Thill M, Fischer D. Epidemiology of vulvar and vaginal cancer in Germany. Arch Gynecol Obstet. 2011;284(1):169–74.
13. Greenstein AJ, Gennuso R, Sachar DB, Heimann T, Smith H, Janowitz HD, et al. Extraintestinal cancers in inflammatory bowel disease. Cancer. 1985;56(12):2914–21.
14. Mir-Madjlessi SH, Farmer RG, Easley KA, Beck GJ. Colorectal and extracolonic malignancy in ulcerative colitis. Cancer. 1986;58(7):1569–74.
15. Jess T, Horvath-Puho E, Fallingborg J, Rasmussen HH, Jacobsen BA. Cancer risk in inflammatory bowel disease according to patient phenotype and treatment: a Danish population-based cohort study. Am J Gastroenterol. 2013;108(12):1869–76.
16. Hemminki K, Liu X, Ji J, Forsti A, Sundquist J, Sundquist K. Effect of autoimmune diseases on risk and survival in female cancers. Gynecol Oncol. 2012;127(1):180–5.
17. Algaba A, Guerra I, Marin-Jimenez I, Quintanilla E, Lopez-Serrano P, Garcia-Sanchez MC, et al. Incidence, management, and course of cancer in patients with inflammatory bowel disease. J Crohns Colitis. 2015;9(4):326–33.
18. Pedersen N, Duricova D, Elkjaer M, Gamborg M, Munkholm P, Jess T. Risk of extra-intestinal cancer in inflammatory bowel disease: meta-analysis of population-based cohort studies. Am J Gastroenterol. 2010;105(7):1480–7.
19. Nyboe Andersen N, Pasternak B, Basit S, Andersson M, Svanstrom H, Caspersen S, et al. Association between tumor necrosis factor-alpha antagonists and risk of cancer in patients with inflammatory bowel disease. JAMA. 2014;311(23):2406–13.
20. Colombel JF, Sands BE, Rutgeerts P, Sandborn W, Danese S, D'Haens G, et al. The safety of vedolizumab for ulcerative colitis and Crohn's disease. Gut. 2017;66(5):839–51.
21. Wang MC, Zhang LY, Han W, Shao Y, Chen M, Ni R, et al. PRISMA – efficacy and safety of vedolizumab for inflammatory bowel diseases: a systematic review and meta-analysis of randomized controlled trials. Medicine (Baltimore). 2014;93(28):e326.
22. Fraser AG, Orchard TR, Robinson EM, Jewell DP. Long-term risk of malignancy after treatment of inflammatory bowel disease with azathioprine. Aliment Pharmacol Ther. 2002;16(7):1225–32.
23. Pasternak B, Svanstrom H, Schmiegelow K, Jess T, Hviid A. Use of azathioprine and the risk of cancer in inflammatory bowel disease. Am J Epidemiol. 2013;177(11):1296–305.
24. Lichtenstein GR, Feagan BG, Cohen RD, Salzberg BA, Diamond RH, Langholff W, et al. Drug therapies and the risk of malignancy in Crohn's disease: results from the TREAT registry. Am J Gastroenterol. 2014;109(2):212–23.
25. Yano Y, Matsui T, Hirai F, Okado Y, Sato Y, Tsurumi K, et al. Cancer risk in Japanese Crohn's disease patients: investigation of the standardized incidence ratio. J Gastroenterol Hepatol. 2013;28(8):1300–5.
26. Fidder H, Schnitzler F, Ferrante M, Noman M, Katsanos K, Segaert S, et al. Long-term safety of infliximab for the treatment of inflammatory bowel disease: a single-centre cohort study. Gut. 2009;58(4):501–8.
27. van den Heuvel TR, Wintjens DS, Jeuring SF, Wassink MH, Romberg-Camps MJ, Oostenbrug LE, et al. Inflammatory bowel disease, cancer and medication: cancer risk in the Dutch population-based IBDSL cohort. Int J Cancer. 2016;139(6):1270–80.
28. Williams CJ, Peyrin-Biroulet L, Ford AC. Systematic review with meta-analysis: malignancies with anti-tumour necrosis factor-alpha therapy in inflammatory bowel disease. Aliment Pharmacol Ther. 2014;39(5):447–58.
29. Armstrong RG, West J, Card TR. Risk of cancer in inflammatory bowel disease treated with azathioprine: a UK population-based case-control study. Am J Gastroenterol. 2010;105(7):1604–9.
30. Siu AL. U.S. preventive services task force. Screening for breast cancer: U.S. preventive services task force recommendation statement. Ann Intern Med. 2016;164(4):279–96.

Chapter 5
Lymphoma Risk and Screening in IBD

Chip Alex Bowman and Garrett Lawlor

Lymphoma in the General Population

The overall incidence of Hodgkin's lymphoma is 2.3/100,000 people/year, carrying a mortality of 0.4 cases/100,000 people/year, with young male adults slightly disproportionately affected and familial clusters suggesting a genetic component [1–3]. Diagnosis is made from excisional lymph node biopsy [1]. Fortunately, with current treatment strategies, 80–90% of diagnosed Hodgkin's lymphoma patients can achieve permanent remission.

Non-Hodgkin's lymphoma (NHL) includes a wide variety of subtypes and is more common in developed regions (Table 5.1) [4]. The incidence rate of NHL rose during the 1990s, but has since stagnated, with an incidence of 19.4 cases/100,000 people/year and a mortality rate of 5.7 cases/100,000 people/year [4–6]. The prior rise is thought to be due to changes in the methods of classification and diagnostic procedures as well as the onset of the AIDS epidemic.

Interestingly, in addition to a predisposition for males, there is also a higher incidence in developed regions compared to the less developed areas for both Hodgkin's lymphoma and NHL.

An increase in the incidence of lymphoma has been associated with chronic inflammatory conditions such as rheumatoid arthritis [3, 7]. Severe disease and the presence of high inflammatory activity were shown to be associated with lymphoma risk, independent of rheumatologic therapies.

C. A. Bowman
Columbia University Vagelos College of Physicians and Surgeons, New York, NY, USA

G. Lawlor (✉)
Columbia University Medical Center/NY-Presbyterian Hospital, New York, NY, USA
e-mail: GL2501@cumc.columbia.edu

© Springer Nature Switzerland AG 2019
J. D. Feuerstein, A. S. Cheifetz (eds.), *Cancer Screening in Inflammatory Bowel Disease*, https://doi.org/10.1007/978-3-030-15301-4_5

Table 5.1 Age-standardized rate (ASR) per 100,000 [4]

	Hodgkin's lymphoma (developed areas)	Hodgkin's lymphoma (less developed areas)	NHL (developed areas)	NHL (less developed areas)
Males	ASR 2.2; mortality 0.4	ASR 0.9; mortality 0.6	ASR 10.3; mortality 3.6	ASR 4.2; mortality 3.0
Females	ASR 1.9; mortality 0.3	ASR 0.5; mortality 0.3	ASR 7.0; mortality 2.2	ASR 2.8; mortality 1.9

Current Screening Strategies for Lymphoma for General and At-Risk Populations

There are currently no screening strategies recommended for lymphoma in patients who are at an average or even high risk, though it is generally recommended to monitor clinically for B-symptoms such as unexplained weight loss, fever, night sweats, or lymphadenopathy [1, 8].

Risk of Lymphoma in IBD

Independent risk factors for lymphoma in IBD patients include increasing age and male gender, which are well-known risk factors in the non-IBD population [9]. While rheumatoid arthritis literature has demonstrated that disease severity is associated with increased risk of lymphoma, evidence that IBD is itself an independent risk factor for lymphoma is conflicting [7, 9].

Multiple large-scale, mostly retrospective, studies have been conducted over the past two decades that attempt to determine the association between IBD and lymphoma risk, but the increasing use of immunosuppressive and biological agents during this time period has confounded the data [3, 10–16]. The current evidence suggests that IBD alone does not independently increase lymphoma risk above that of the general population, though the data remains overall contradictory [10, 11, 17–20]. Heterogeneous publications with underpowered and differing population demographics and often under-reporting of therapies employed may reflect varied risk rates [10, 21]. Ignoring for a moment the impact of medications on lymphoma risk in the IBD population, the increased overall risk of lymphoma in the elderly population can lead to a reasonable recommendation that special attention be given to potential signs of lymphoma in the older IBD population [8, 22].

IBD Therapy and Lymphoma

Inflammatory bowel disease management has evolved over the years, and while efficacious, some therapies raise concerns over their independent risk of malignancy including the development of lymphoma. Immunosuppression has long been shown to be associated with increased risk of lymphoproliferative disorders such as non-Hodgkin's lymphoma, though the dosages are often lower in IBD typically than in established risk pools such as in post-transplant patients, and as such the risk may be slightly lower [3, 20]. As the use of immunosuppressive agents and biologics increases in the management of IBD, balancing the risks and benefits of medical therapy becomes more prudent, especially regarding the risks of long-term therapy. In general, this has been a difficult area of study due to small cohorts in prospective analyses and teasing out risk in patients with a history of exposure to multiple classes of medications [23]. This section will summarize the current data on lymphoma risk in IBD for each of the major immunosuppressive therapies.

Thiopurines: Azathioprine (AZA) and 6-Mercaptopurine (6-MP)

Thiopurines were first demonstrated in the 1970s to have an association with non-Hodgkin's lymphoma development in post-kidney transplant studies, and the association was later shown in the 2000s to be also seen with IBD treatment [2]. Azathioprine/6-mercaptopurine (AZA/6-MP) are purine analogues that interfere with nucleic acid metabolism and thus dampen the immune response; as such, they are used to maintain remission in Crohn's disease and ulcerative colitis [3, 24, 25]. Many cases of thiopurine-associated lymphoproliferative cancers are associated with EBV virus, discussed in greater detail below.

While there are multiple studies investigating lymphoma risk with thiopurines, many of these studies are limited in their generalizability and confounding by indication [26]. Furthermore, conflicting data has been published regarding long-term use of thiopurine therapy in IBD patients and the subsequent development of lymphoma [27]. AZA and 6-MP have demonstrated association of developing lymphoma with increased risk in IBD patients in addition to prolonging life expectancy, though the absolute increase in lymphoma risk is low [19, 24].

Because IBD is a chronic and incurable disease, long-term therapy with these agents may have an added effect on risk. Though the lymphoma risk with thiopurines does not appear to become clinically apparent until after at least 1 year of use, it continues to increase over the long term [23, 28]. Khan et al. suggest at least a fourfold increase in risk in UC patients receiving thiopurine therapy compared with those not on immunosuppression, which increases over time and as such is a limiting factor in prolonged thiopurine therapy [29–32]. Importantly, discontinuation of thiopurine therapy appears to lead to normalization of lymphoma risk [30, 32, 33].

Anti-TNF

When first approved by the FDA in 1998, there were no incident reports of lymphoma for infliximab in Crohn's disease patients, which was promptly supported by retrospective studies and the first prospective trial [26]. There remained a lingering concern regarding lymphoma risk with anti-TNF supported by even recent studies [34], and by 2002, the FDA's adverse event surveillance system documented "possible" or "probable" infliximab-associated lymphoma cases, and in 2004, lymphoma risk was added to the packaging insert [26].

Over time, multiple studies assessing the safety profile of adalimumab in Crohn's disease demonstrated no increased risk for lymphoma development in IBD or rheumatoid arthritis patients [9, 35–40]. It was considered that lymphoma risk could possibly be attributed to disease severity rather than TNF-alpha treatment exposure [41]. Although the safety profile is generally favorable, high-risk individuals such as those with known malignancy or prior lymphoma warrant close monitoring [42]. Following from this, a meta-analysis by Siegel et al. published in 2009 did conclude a slightly increased lymphoma risk with anti-TNF agents with a standardized incident rate ratio (SIRR) of 3.23 (95% CI 1.5–6.9), though again most patients had prior thiopurine exposure [43].

In more recent times, anti-TNF therapy has been demonstrated in multiple studies to have comparable rates of risk of lymphoma as the treatment-naive population and has an overall good safety profile [44–49]. The TREAT Registry (Crohn's Therapy, Resource, Evaluation, and Assessment Tool), a large prospectively enrolled cohort study of 6273 patients with Crohn's disease, showed increased risk of malignancy with age, disease duration, and smoking, but not with infliximab [50]. Of note, TREAT also found no significant impact of thiopurine use on lymphoma risk.

Combination Therapy (Anti-TNF and Thiopurines)

In the current climate of combination therapy of thiopurine and biological therapies in the treatment of IBD, optimized use of these drugs in a safe and effective manner is vital. As discussed above, safety from a lymphoma perspective appears to be a concern after at least 1 year on thiopurines. From an efficacy standpoint, retrospective data suggest there may be a limit to duration of efficacy of thiopurines in the setting of combination therapy. Drobne et al. noted in retrospective data that thiopurine utility wanes after 6 months of combination therapy [51]. Thus, dose optimization of biological therapy may negate the need for continued thiopurine use after 1 year. With that in mind, what is the risk of lymphoma in the combination therapy patient?

Herrington et al.'s 2011 retrospective analysis of 16,023 IBD patients within the Kaiser Permanente IBD Registry noted that the use of anti-TNF with thiopurines in addition to monotherapy with thiopurines were associated with an increased risk of lymphoma, with a standardized incidence rate ratio (SIRR) of 5.5 in TNF-exposed patients, of whom most (85%) had concomitant or previous thiopurine exposure [28]. In 2017, Lemaitre et al. published in *JAMA* a French nationwide cohort study of 189,289 patients of whom 14,229 were exposed to both anti-TNF and thiopurines – adjusted hazard ratio (aHR) for lymphoma with combination therapy was

6.11 compared to 2.60 for thiopurine monotherapy or 2.41 for anti-TNF mono-therapy [52, 53]. As such combination therapy of thiopurine and anti-TNF carries the highest risk for lymphoma over monotherapy of either agent [40].

Newer Agents

In recent years, the FDA has approved a number of therapies with novel targets in the management of IBD. Vedolizumab, ustekinumab, and tofacitinib have not dem-onstrated significant safety signals for lymphoma and as such may be preferred in patients who are considered to be at high risk for lymphoma. Please see chap. 8 Cancer Risks and Screening with Current and Emerging Drug Therapies in Inflammatory Bowel Diseases for a further in depth review of the risks of lym-phoma with current and emerging drug therapies in inflammatory bowel disease.

Epstein-Barr Virus-Associated Lymphomas

The Epstein-Barr virus (EBV) is a human herpes virus whose reservoir are B-cell lymphocytes. Lymphoproliferative disorders, such as NHL, associated with EBV have been shown to occur in immunocompromised patients, such as post-transplant patients that comprise the main sample population for this subset of data in the lit-erature [3]. The vast majority of non-Hodgkin's lymphomas that occur in post-transplant patients have been associated with EBV infection. High EBV viral load was found to show increased risk of NHL in the transplant setting [54, 55].

Thiopurine-associated lymphomas have been recorded with EBV-associated B-cell lymphoma, a rare yet often fatal form of lymphoma [2, 19, 23, 30, 56–58]. It is thought that in these patients, who convert to seropositive for EBV while on such therapy, non-Hodgkin's lymphoma is attributed to the thiopurine cytotoxic effects on EBV-specific immune cells. Reactivation of chronic latent EBV infection is associated with post-transplant-like lymphomas in IBD adults treated with thiopu-rines [59]. The CESAME cohort study noted an increased risk in developing EBV-positive lymphoma when patients are receiving thiopurines that reduces to treatment-naïve levels when thiopurines are discontinued [26]. As such, populations highest at risk, such as young men seronegative for EBV upon initiation of therapy, may have increased risk of developing lymphoma after developing acute infectious mononucleosis in the setting of a thiopurine [30]. It may thus be reasonable to screen for EBV before initiating thiopurines, irrespective of sex or age, and poten-tially avoid thiopurines in EBV-negative cohorts [60, 61]. Additionally, regular quantitative monitoring of EBV reactivation coupled with pre-emptive rituximab therapy has been considered an effective strategy to improve outcomes in patients at high risk of EBV-related lymphoma (specifically after allogeneic stem cell trans-plantation) [62, 63].

Hepatosplenic T-Cell Lymphoma: Peculiar to IBD Management

Hepatosplenic T-cell lymphoma (HSTCL) is a rare type of lymphoma (<5% of T-cell lymphomas) in which atypical lymphocytes infiltrate the splenic red pulp and intrasinusoidal space in the liver and bone marrow. Patients present with hepatosplenomegaly, blood dyscrasias, and liver enzyme abnormalities in the absence of lymphadenopathy [64]. HSTCL carries a high mortality and demonstrates an overrepresentation of IBD patients contributing to the data, particularly men between the ages of 15 and 40 [65].

The increasing use of immunosuppression and biological therapies in patients with IBD appear to be affecting this trend [26, 65–67]. In 2009, Kotlyar et al. published a systematic review of HSTCL in the setting of anti-TNF and thiopurine therapies, demonstrating that long-term therapy of at least 2 years of thiopurines as monotherapy or combined therapy with anti-TNF in young men merits monitoring for HSTCL or should be recommended to avoid thiopurines due to the increased risk [30, 65].

Data available on the FDA Adverse Events Reporting System (FDAERS) database provides some insight into the occurrence of HSTCL in IBD patients (Table 5.2) [68]. A total of 226 cases with 137 deaths have been recorded to date (September 2018) in the database that was first recorded in 2002. Demographic data shows that 64% of cases were in males and 23% in females (gender unrecorded in the remainder). Of those that had a recorded age, the majority took place between the ages of 18 and 64 (84%).

Of the 226 reported cases of HSCTL, 147 were in IBD patients, of which 122 had Crohn's disease and 25 had ulcerative colitis. Indeterminate cases are those whose diagnosis was not definitive in the FDA database. Age range was wide – 12–81 years in Crohn's disease (median 30 years) and 16–70 years in ulcerative colitis (median 27 years). The proportion of male patients was 88% in Crohn's disease and 26% in ulcerative colitis for data that was reported (not including unreported data from 19 subjects).

There is reported increased risk of HSTCL with some therapies commonly used in IBD regimens (Figs. 5.1 and 5.2). Deepak et al. in 2013 published data comparing FDAERS data to the SEER 17 registry and noted an increased risk of T-cell NHL in combination therapy and thiopurine monotherapy, but not in anti-TNF monotherapy [69, 70]. This is in consensus with other findings that suggest that thiopurines, whether in monotherapy or combination therapy, are the main drivers for HSTCL in IBD patients, particularly in young males [65, 71, 72]. Overall, the rarity of HSTCL and the possibility of under-reporting to FDAERS make it difficult to assess the true risk of HSTCL with each therapy.

Table 5.2 FDAERS database reported HSTCL cases in IBD patients from 2002 to 2018

	Sex				Age			Drug				Mortality	
	Male	Female	Unrecorded	Total	Minimum	Median	Maximum	Thiopurine	Anti-TNF	Anti-TNF + thiopurine therapy	Other	Survived	Died
Non-IBD/unclear	44	24	11	79	15	30	77	20	26	26	7	34	45
IBD	101	27	19	147	12	29	81	26	32	78	11	55	92
Total	145	51	30	226				46	58	104	18	89	137
CD	96	13	13	122	12	30	81	24	16	74	8	38	84
Indeterminate	14	12	2	28	15	51	70	7	14	4	3	14	14
Not IBD	30	12	9	51	16	27	77	13	12	22	4	20	31
UC	5	14	6	25	16	27	70	2	16	4	3	17	8
Total	145	51	30	226				46	58	104	18	89	137

CD Crohn's disease, *UC* ulcerative colitis

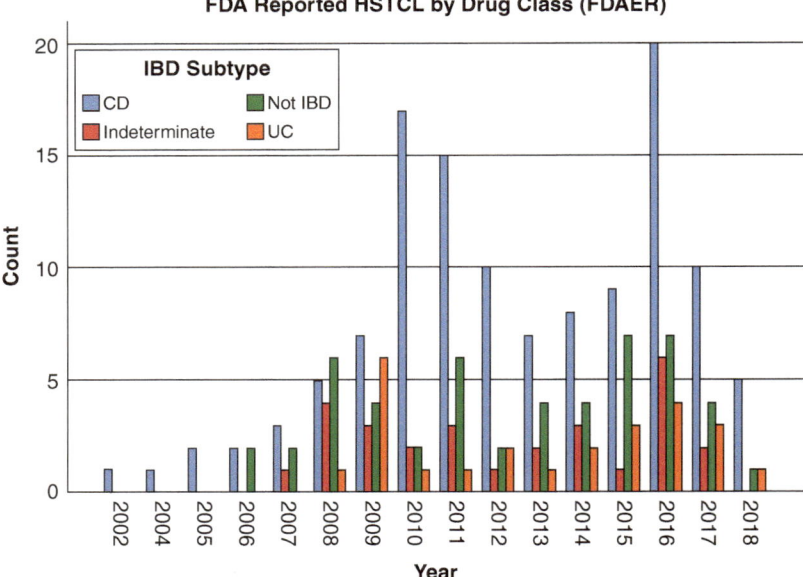

Fig. 5.1 FDAER data of HSTCL cases reported by year, by IBD subtype

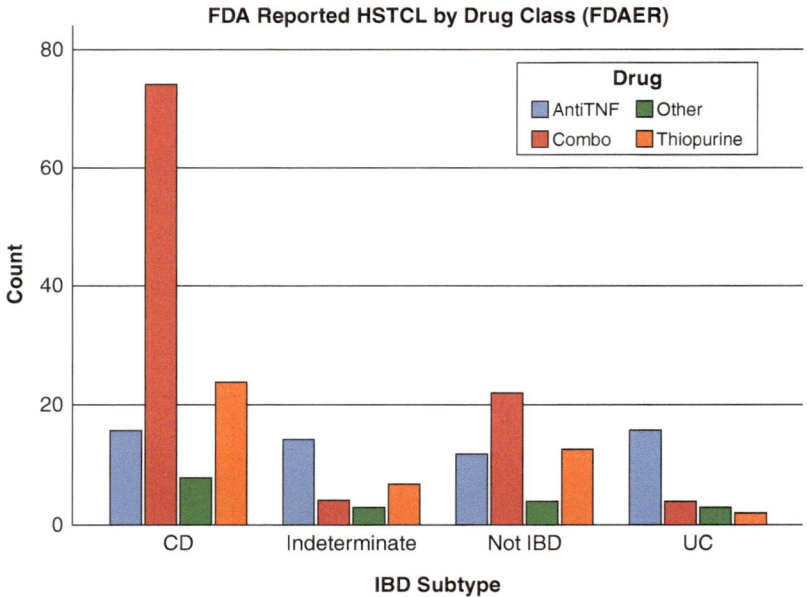

Fig. 5.2 FDAER data of HSTCL in IBD patients by drug class

Pediatric Experience

Pediatric-onset IBD is associated with a more severe disease phenotype; as such, there has been a growing concern regarding lymphoma risk – especially for patients on thiopurines [73]. Two systematic reviews have been more recently published that summarize the lymphoma risk on biological therapy [37, 73]. Dulai et al. published in systematic analysis an absolute rate of lymphoma of 2.1/10,000 person-years based on two reported cases, both exposed to combination therapy [69]. More recently, Hyams et al. collected and analyzed data from 5766 pediatric participants in a prospective study from 2007 to 2016, reporting five cases of lymphoma [47]. Three of the five were exposed to anti-TNF, four were exposed to thiopurines, also suggesting a greater role of thiopurine monotherapy or combination therapy (thiopurine and anti-TNF) in the development of lymphoma in children.

High-Risk Population: Prior Lymphoma

As IBD is a lifelong disease that affects young people, there is concern for new and recurrent cancer risk throughout a patient's lifetime, especially as immunosuppressant therapies may promote several types of cancers [74]. There is very little data to guide us on the safety of anti-TNF and thiopurines in patients with previous lymphoma [75, 76]. Current prospective studies are underway to determine this safety issue.

Key Points
1. The weight of literature suggests that IBD is not in itself an independent risk factor for lymphoma development.
2. There is currently no recommended screening strategy for lymphoma in the IBD population, though concerning symptoms such as unexplained weight loss and fevers should be investigated for possible underlying lymphoma.
3. Use of a thiopurine for cumulatively less than 1 year does not appear to increase lymphoma risk.
4. Thiopurines use for over 2 years appears to increase lymphoma risk fourfold in IBD patients, and this risk may increase further with longer-term use.
5. The risk of lymphoma reverts to that of the general population when the thiopurine is discontinued for greater than a year.
6. Anti-TNF therapy in IBD does not appear to impact lymphoma risk, though the data is not entirely clear. For this reason, we would still recommend avoiding anti-TNF therapies in patients with a prior personal history of lymphoma.
7. Combination of thiopurine and anti-TNF therapy increases lymphoma risk more than thiopurine monotherapy or anti-TNF monotherapy.
8. There may be rationale to avoid thiopurines in patients who are EBV-negative to avoid the development of NHL in the setting of EBV seroconversion.
9. Young men may be at particular risk of HSTCL in the setting of thiopurine use (and possibly anti-TNF); thus, it may be prudent to avoid in this population.

References

1. Eichenauer DA, Engert A, André M, et al. Hodgkin's lymphoma: ESMO clinical practice guidelines for diagnosis, treatment and follow-up. Ann Oncol. 2014;25:iii70–i5.
2. Beaugerie L, Itzkowitz SH. Cancers complicating inflammatory bowel disease. N Engl J Med. 2015;372:1441–52.
3. Sokol H, Beaugerie L. Inflammatory bowel disease and lymphoproliferative disorders: the dust is starting to settle. Gut. 2009;58:1427–36.
4. Jemal A, Bray F, Center MM, Ferlay J, Ward E, Forman D. Global cancer statistics. CA Cancer J Clin. 2011;61:69–90.
5. Horesh N, Horowitz NA. Does gender matter in non-Hodgkin lymphoma? Differences in epidemiology, clinical behavior, and therapy. Rambam Maimonides Med J. 2014;5:e0038.
6. Cancer stat facts: non-Hodgkin lymphoma. seer.cancer.gov. Accessed 9 Oct 2018.
7. Baecklund E, Iliadou A, Askling J, et al. Association of chronic inflammation, not its treatment, with increased lymphoma risk in rheumatoid arthritis. Arthritis Rheum. 2006;54:692–701.
8. Taleban S, Elquza E, Gower-Rousseau C, Peyrin-Biroulet L. Cancer and inflammatory bowel disease in the elderly. Dig Liver Dis. 2016;48:1105–11.
9. Afif W, Sandborn WJ, Faubion WA, et al. Risk factors for lymphoma in patients with inflammatory bowel disease: a case-control study. Inflamm Bowel Dis. 2013;19:1384–9.
10. Kappelman MD, Farkas DK, Long MD, et al. Risk of cancer in patients with inflammatory bowel diseases: a nationwide population-based cohort study with 30 years of follow-up evaluation. Clin Gastroenterol Hepatol. 2014;12:265–73.e1.
11. Garg SK, Velayos FS, Kisiel JB. Intestinal and nonintestinal cancer risks for patients with Crohn's disease. Gastroenterol Clin. 2017;46:515–29.
12. Jones JL, Loftus EV Jr. Lymphoma risk in inflammatory bowel disease: is it the disease or its treatment? Inflamm Bowel Dis. 2007;13:1299–307.
13. Farrell R, Ang Y, Kileen P, et al. Increased incidence of non-Hodgkin's lymphoma in inflammatory bowel disease patients on immunosuppressive therapy but overall risk is low. Gut. 2000;47:514–9.
14. Lewis JD, Bilker WB, Brensinger C, Deren JJ, Vaughn DJ, Strom BL. Inflammatory bowel disease is not associated with an increased risk of lymphoma. Gastroenterology. 2001;121:1080–7.
15. Loftus EV Jr, Tremaine WJ, Habermann TM, Harmsen WS, Zinsmeister AR, Sandborn WJ. Risk of lymphoma in inflammatory bowel disease. Am J Gastroenterol. 2000;95:2308.
16. Greenstein AJ, Mullin GE, Strauchen JA, et al. Lymphoma in inflammatory bowel disease. Cancer. 1992;69:1119–23.
17. Garg SK, Loftus EV. Risk of cancer in inflammatory bowel disease: going up, going down, or still the same? Curr Opin Gastroenterol. 2016;32:274–81.
18. van den Heuvel TR, Wintjens DS, Jeuring SF, et al. Inflammatory bowel disease, cancer and medication: cancer risk in the Dutch population-based IBDSL cohort. Int J Cancer. 2016;139:1270–80.
19. Vos A, Bakkal N, Minnee R, et al. Risk of malignant lymphoma in patients with inflammatory bowel diseases: a Dutch nationwide study. Inflamm Bowel Dis. 2011;17:1837–45.
20. Kwon JH, Farrell RJ. The risk of lymphoma in the treatment of inflammatory bowel disease with immunosuppressive agents. Crit Rev Oncol Hematol. 2005;56:169–78.
21. Wheat CL, Clark-Snustad K, Devine B, Grembowski D, Thornton TA, Ko CW. Worldwide incidence of colorectal cancer, leukemia, and lymphoma in inflammatory bowel disease: an updated systematic review and meta-analysis. Gastroenterol Res Pract. 2016;2016:1632439.
22. Shrestha MP, Ruel J, Taleban S. Healthcare maintenance in elderly patients with inflammatory bowel disease. Ann Gastroenterol. 2017;30:273.
23. Mason M, Siegel CA. Do inflammatory bowel disease therapies cause cancer? Inflamm Bowel Dis. 2013;19:1306–21.
24. Lewis JD, Schwartz JS, Lichtenstein GR. Azathioprine for maintenance of remission in Crohn's disease: benefits outweigh the risk of lymphoma. Gastroenterology. 2000;118:1018–24.

25. Chande N, Patton PH, Tsoulis DJ, Thomas BS, MacDonald JK. Azathioprine or 6-mercaptopurine for maintenance of remission in Crohn's disease. 2015.
26. Bewtra M, Lewis JD. Update on the risk of lymphoma following immunosuppressive therapy for inflammatory bowel disease. Expert Rev Clin Immunol. 2010;6:621–31.
27. McGovern DP, Travis SP. Thiopurine therapy: when to start and when to stop. Eur J Gastroenterol Hepatol. 2003;15:219–23.
28. Herrinton LJ, Liu L, Weng X, Lewis JD, Hutfless S, Allison JE. Role of thiopurine and anti-TNF therapy in lymphoma in inflammatory bowel disease. Am J Gastroenterol. 2011;106:2146.
29. Kandiel A, Fraser A, Korelitz B, Brensinger C, Lewis J. Increased risk of lymphoma among inflammatory bowel disease patients treated with azathioprine and 6-mercaptopurine. Gut. 2005;54:1121–5.
30. Swoger JM, Regueiro M. Stopping, continuing, or restarting immunomodulators and biologics when an infection or malignancy develops. Inflamm Bowel Dis. 2014;20:926–35.
31. Beaugerie L, Brousse N, Bouvier AM, et al. Lymphoproliferative disorders in patients receiving thiopurines for inflammatory bowel disease: a prospective observational cohort study. Lancet. 2009;374:1617–25.
32. Khan N, Abbas AM, Lichtenstein GR, Loftus EV Jr, Bazzano LA. Risk of lymphoma in patients with ulcerative colitis treated with thiopurines: a nationwide retrospective cohort study. Gastroenterology. 2013;145:1007–15.e3.
33. Kotlyar DS, Lewis JD, Beaugerie L, et al. Risk of lymphoma in patients with inflammatory bowel disease treated with azathioprine and 6-mercaptopurine: a meta-analysis. Clin Gastroenterol Hepatol. 2015;13:847–58.e4.
34. Hansen RA, Gartlehner G, Powell GE, Sandler RS. Serious adverse events with infliximab: analysis of spontaneously reported adverse events. Clin Gastroenterol Hepatol. 2007;5:729–35.
35. D'Haens G, Reinisch W, Panaccione R, et al. Lymphoma risk and overall safety profile of adalimumab in patients with Crohn's disease with up to 6 years of follow-up in the pyramid registry. Am J Gastroenterol. 2018;1:872–82.
36. Andersen NN, Pasternak B, Basit S, et al. Association between tumor necrosis factor-α antagonists and risk of cancer in patients with inflammatory bowel disease. JAMA. 2014;311:2406–13.
37. Dulai PS, Thompson KD, Blunt HB, Dubinsky MC, Siegel CA. Risks of serious infection or lymphoma with anti-tumor necrosis factor therapy for pediatric inflammatory bowel disease: a systematic review. Clin Gastroenterol Hepatol. 2014;12:1443–51.
38. Williams CJ, Peyrin-Biroulet L, Ford AC. Systematic review with meta-analysis: malignancies with anti-tumour necrosis factor-alpha therapy in inflammatory bowel disease. Aliment Pharmacol Ther. 2014;39:447–58.
39. Kopylov U, Vutcovici M, Kezouh A, Seidman E, Bitton A, Afif W. Risk of lymphoma, colorectal and skin cancer in patients with IBD treated with immunomodulators and biologics: a Quebec claims database study. Inflamm Bowel Dis. 2015;21:1847–53.
40. Dassopoulos T, Sultan S, Falck-Ytter YT, Inadomi JM, Hanauer SB. American Gastroenterological Association Institute technical review on the use of thiopurines, methotrexate, and anti-TNF-α biologic drugs for the induction and maintenance of remission in inflammatory Crohn's disease. Gastroenterology. 2013;145:1464–78.e5.
41. Chen Y, Friedman M, Liu G, Deodhar A, Chu C-Q. Do tumor necrosis factor inhibitors increase cancer risk in patients with chronic immune-mediated inflammatory disorders? Cytokine. 2018;101:78–88.
42. Van Assche G, Lewis JD, Lichtenstein GR, et al. The London position statement of the world congress of gastroenterology on biological therapy for IBD with the European Crohn's and colitis organisation: safety. Am J Gastroenterol. 2011;106:1594.
43. Siegel CA, Marden SM, Persing SM, Larson RJ, Sands BE. Risk of lymphoma associated with combination anti-tumor necrosis factor and immunomodulator therapy for the treatment of Crohn's disease: a meta-analysis. Clin Gastroenterol Hepatol. 2009;7:874–81.
44. Biancone L, Orlando A, Kohn A, et al. Infliximab and newly diagnosed neoplasia in Crohn's disease: a multicentre matched pair study. Gut. 2006;55:228–33.

45. Biancone L, Petruzziello C, Orlando A, et al. Cancer in Crohn's disease patients treated with infliximab: a long-term multicenter matched pair study. Inflamm Bowel Dis. 2010;17:758–66.
46. Fidder H, Schnitzler F, Ferrante M, et al. Long-term safety of infliximab for the treatment of inflammatory bowel disease: a single-centre cohort study. Gut. 2009;58:501–8.
47. Hyams JS, Dubinsky MC, Baldassano RN, et al. Infliximab is not associated with increased risk of malignancy or hemophagocytic lymphohistiocytosis in pediatric patients with inflammatory bowel disease. Gastroenterology. 2017;152:1901–14.e3.
48. Miehsler W, Novacek G, Wenzl H, et al. A decade of infliximab: the Austrian evidence based consensus on the safe use of infliximab in inflammatory bowel disease. J Crohn's Colitis. 2010;4:221–56.
49. Caspersen S, Elkjaer M, Riis L, et al. Infliximab for inflammatory bowel disease in Denmark 1999–2005: clinical outcome and follow-up evaluation of malignancy and mortality. Clin Gastroenterol Hepatol. 2008;6:1212–7.
50. Lichtenstein GR, Feagan BG, Cohen RD, et al. Drug therapies and the risk of malignancy in Crohn's disease: results from the TREAT™ registry. Am J Gastroenterol. 2014;109:212.
51. Drobne D, Bossuyt P, Breynaert C, et al. Withdrawal of immunomodulators after co-treatment does not reduce trough level of infliximab in patients with Crohn's disease. Clin Gastroenterol Hepatol. 2015;13:514–21.e4.
52. Targownik LE, Bernstein CN. Infectious and malignant complications of TNF inhibitor therapy in IBD. Am J Gastroenterol. 2013;108:1835.
53. Lemaitre M, Kirchgesner J, Rudnichi A, et al. Association between use of thiopurines or tumor necrosis factor antagonists alone or in combination and risk of lymphoma in patients with inflammatory bowel disease. JAMA. 2017;318:1679–86.
54. Reijasse D, Le Pendeven C, Cosnes J, et al. Epstein-Barr virus viral load in Crohn's disease: effect of immunosuppressive therapy. Inflamm Bowel Dis. 2004;10:85–90.
55. Stevens SJ, Verschuuren EA, Pronk I, et al. Frequent monitoring of Epstein-Barr virus DNA load in unfractionated whole blood is essential for early detection of posttransplant lymphoproliferative disease in high-risk patients. Blood. 2001;97:1165–71.
56. Dayharsh GA, Loftus EV Jr, Sandborn WJ, et al. Epstein-Barr virus-positive lymphoma in patients with inflammatory bowel disease treated with azathioprine or 6-mercaptopurine. Gastroenterology. 2002;122:72–7.
57. Serrate C, Silva-Moreno M, Dartigues P, et al. Epstein-Barr virus-associated lymphoproliferation awareness in hemophagocytic syndrome complicating thiopurine treatment for Crohn's disease. Inflamm Bowel Dis. 2009;15:1449–51.
58. Virdis F, Tacci S, Messina F, Varcada M. Hemophagocytic lymphohistiocytosis caused by primary Epstein-Barr virus in patient with Crohn's disease. World J Gastrointest Surg. 2013;5:306–8.
59. Münz C, Moormann A. Immune escape by Epstein-Barr virus associated malignancies. Semin Cancer Biol. 2008;18:381–7. Elsevier.
60. Gordon J, Ramaswami A, Beuttler M, et al. EBV status and thiopurine use in pediatric IBD. J Pediatr Gastroenterol Nutr. 2016;62:711–4.
61. Biank VF, Sheth MK, Talano J, et al. Association of Crohn's disease, thiopurines, and primary Epstein-Barr virus infection with hemophagocytic lymphohistiocytosis. J Pediatr. 2011;159:808–12.
62. van Esser JW, Niesters HG, van der Holt B, et al. Prevention of Epstein-Barr virus-lymphoproliferative disease by molecular monitoring and preemptive rituximab in high-risk patients after allogeneic stem cell transplantation. Blood. 2002;99:4364–9.
63. Weinstock D, Ambrossi G, Brennan C, Kiehn T, Jakubowski A. Preemptive diagnosis and treatment of Epstein-Barr virus-associated post transplant lymphoproliferative disorder after hematopoietic stem cell transplant: an approach in development. Bone Marrow Transplant. 2006;37:539.
64. Thai A, Prindiville T. Hepatosplenic T-cell lymphoma and inflammatory bowel disease. J Crohn's Colitis. 2010;4:511–22.

65. Kotlyar DS, Osterman MT, Diamond RH, et al. A systematic review of factors that contribute to hepatosplenic T-cell lymphoma in patients with inflammatory bowel disease. Clin Gastroenterol Hepatol. 2011;9:36–41.e1.
66. Shale M, Kanfer E, Panaccione R, Ghosh S. Hepatosplenic T-cell lymphoma in inflammatory bowel disease. Gut. 2008;57:1639.
67. Mekelburg S, Schneider Y, Pizzi M, Chadburn A, Mathew S. The risk of hepatosplenic T-cell lymphoma (HSTCL) in women with inflammatory bowel disease (IBD) on thiopurines. J Inflam Bowel Dis Disord. 2016;1:110; 3:3
68. FDA. Hepatosplenic T-cell lymphoma. FDA adverse events reporting system (FAERS) 2018.
69. Dulai PS, Siegel CA. The risk of malignancy associated with the use of biological agents in patients with inflammatory bowel disease. Gastroenterol Clin. 2014;43:525–41.
70. Deepak P, Sifuentes H, Sherid M, Stobaugh D, Sadozai Y, Ehrenpreis ED. T-cell non-Hodgkin's lymphomas reported to the FDA AERS with tumor necrosis factor-alpha (TNF-α) inhibitors: results of the REFURBISH study. Am J Gastroenterol. 2013;108:99.
71. Rosh JR, Gross T, Mamula P, Griffiths A, Hyams J. Hepatosplenic T-cell lymphoma in adolescents and young adults with Crohn's disease: a cautionary tale? Inflamm Bowel Dis. 2007;13:1024–30.
72. Dulai PS, Siegel CA, Colombel J-F, Sandborn WJ, Peyrin-Biroulet L. Systematic review: monotherapy with antitumour necrosis factor α agents versus combination therapy with an immunosuppressive for IBD. Gut. 2014;63:1843–53.
73. Aardoom MA, Joosse ME, de Vries ACH, Levine A, de Ridder L. Malignancy and mortality in pediatric-onset inflammatory bowel disease: a systematic review. Inflamm Bowel Dis. 2018;24:732–41.
74. Bernheim O, Colombel J-F, Ullman TA, Laharie D, Beaugerie L, Itzkowitz SH. The management of immunosuppression in patients with inflammatory bowel disease and cancer. Gut. 2013;62:1523–8.
75. Axelrad J, Bernheim O, Colombel J-F, et al. Risk of new or recurrent cancer in patients with inflammatory bowel disease and previous cancer exposed to immunosuppressive and anti-tumor necrosis factor agents. Clin Gastroenterol Hepatol. 2016;14:58–64.
76. Beaugerie L, Carrat F, Colombel J-F, et al. Risk of new or recurrent cancer under immunosuppressive therapy in patients with IBD and previous cancer. Gut. 2014;63:1416–23.

Chapter 6
Pouch Neoplasia Following IPAA in Patients with Underlying Inflammatory Bowel Diseases

Freeha Khan and Bo Shen

Abbreviations

ATZ   Anal transitional zone
CAN   Colitis-associated neoplasia
CD   Crohn's disease
CRC   Colorectal cancer
EMR   Endoscopic mucosal resection
HGD   High-grade dysplasia
IBD   Inflammatory bowel disease
IND   Indefinite for dysplasia
IPAA   Ileal pouch-anal anastomosis
LGD   Low-grade dysplasia
PSC   Primary sclerosing cholangitis
UC   Ulcerative colitis

Introduction

Restorative proctocolectomy with ileal pouch-anal anastomosis (IPAA) is the gold standard surgical treatment of choice for colitis-associated neoplasia, medically refractory ulcerative colitis (UC), and familial adenomatous polyposis. IPAA markedly improves patients' quality of life by avoiding the need for lifelong ileostomy and retaining the natural route of defecation. Promising functional outcomes of

F. Khan · B. Shen (✉)
Center for Inflammatory Bowel Disease, Digestive Disease and Surgery Institute-A31,
Cleveland Clinic, Cleveland, OH, USA
e-mail: shenb@ccf.org

© Springer Nature Switzerland AG 2019
J. D. Feuerstein, A. S. Cheifetz (eds.), *Cancer Screening in Inflammatory Bowel Disease*, https://doi.org/10.1007/978-3-030-15301-4_6

IPAA have been reported by long-term follow-up studies [1–3]. However, the risk for neoplasia of the pouch may still exist, despite the removal of the diseased colon. Pouch neoplasia is defined as the presence of histologic evidence on endoscopic or surgical specimen of low-grade dysplasia (LGD), high-grade dysplasia (HGD), or colorectal cancer (CRC) at the anal transitional zone (ATZ) or cuff, or less often in the pouch body or afferent limb. A combined clinical, endoscopic, and histologic examination plays an essential role in diagnosis and management. Routine surveillance pouchoscopy is recommended in those at risk.

Incidence and Prevalence of Pouch Dysplasia

The reported cumulative prevalence of pouch neoplasia ranges from 0% up to 18.5% [4–9]. Our recent study of 3203 patients with ileal pouches showed that the cumulative incidence for pouch neoplasia at 5, 10, 15, 20, and 25 years after pouch construction was 0.9%, 1.3%, 1.9%, 4.2%, and 5.1%, respectively [10]. A Dutch pathology registry identified 1200 patients with inflammatory bowel disease (IBD) and IPAA from January 1991 to May 2012. The investigators found that 25 (1.83%) developed pouch neoplasia, including 16 adenocarcinomas. Furthermore, cumulative incidences of pouch neoplasia and pouch carcinoma at 5, 10, 15, and 20 years were 1.0%, 2.0%, 3.7%, and 6.9% and 0.6%, 1.4%, 2.1%, and 3.3%, respectively [11].

Risk Factors

The exact pathogenesis of pouch-associated neoplasia is not clear. The main risk factor for pouch neoplasia is a preoperative diagnosis of UC-associated dysplasia or the presence of CAN before or at the time of colectomy [10, 12]. The presence of precolectomy colon dysplasia or CRC is associated with an estimated 4- and 25-fold increase in risk, respectively, of developing pouch neoplasia [11]. Other purported risk factors include concurrent primary sclerosing cholangitis (PSC), the presence of type C mucosa of the pouch, a family history of CRC, and a long duration of underlying UC [13]. Chronic pouch inflammation, such as chronic pouchitis, Crohn's disease (CD) of the pouch, or chronic refractory cuffitis, may increase the risk for the development of neoplasia.

Clinical Presentation of Pouch Neoplasia

Patients with pouch neoplasia can be totally asymptomatic. Patients usually present with symptoms such as diarrhea or abdominal cramps from concurrent pouchitis, CD of the pouch, or cuffitis [14]. Systemic manifestations, such as fever, anemia, or weight loss are rare. However, there are no specific symptoms associated with pouch neoplasia.

Endoscopic Features of Pouch Neoplasia

Pouchoscopy with biopsy remains the gold standard for the early detection and diagnosis of pouch neoplasia. Common endoscopic features include ulcerated lesions, polypoid lesions, adenocarcinoma, or flat dysplasia in the cuff (Fig. 6.1) [15]. It is recommended to remove large, such as more than 1 cm, polypoid lesions of the pouch or ATZ to rule out neoplasia (Fig. 6.2). Previous studies reported that 8.7% (2 of 23) of those polyps were found to be neoplastic [15]. Some patients, however, may not have endoscopic visible lesion. This is particularly true in those with mucosectomy and handsewn anastomosis for precolectomy CAN.

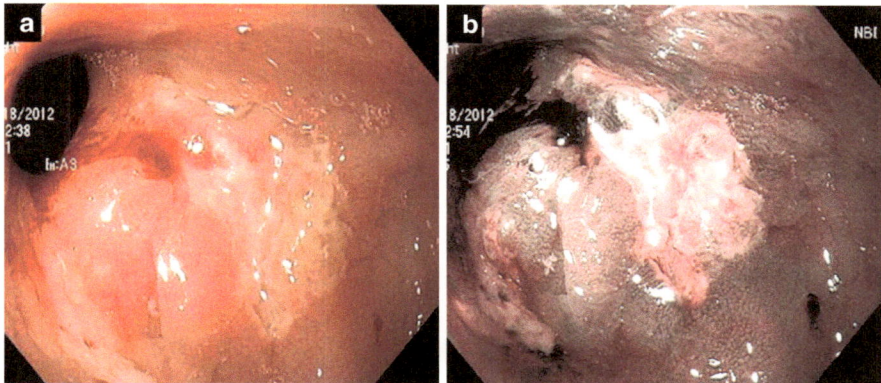

Fig. 6.1 White light (**a**) and narrow-band imaging in the detection of flat dysplasia in the cuff (**b**)

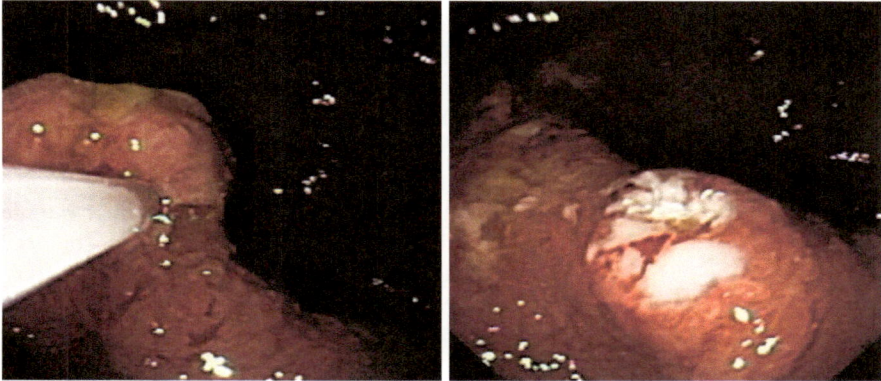

Fig. 6.2 Endoscopic polypectomy in a patient with distal pouch polyp

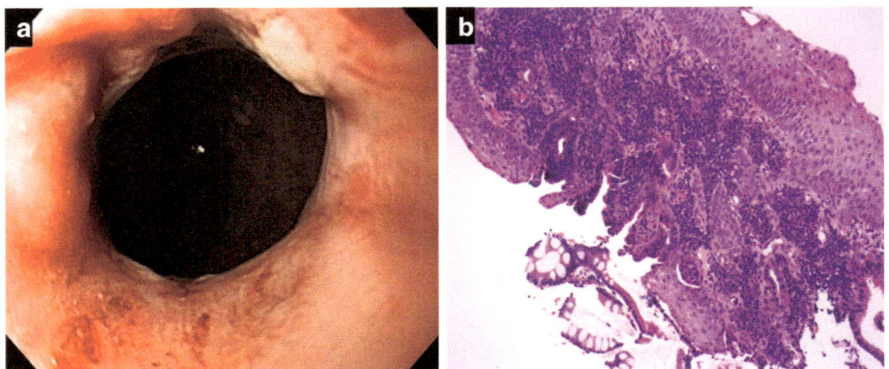

Fig. 6.3 Pouch cancer. Unremarkable anal transitional zone (**a**); deep biopsy showing cancer underneath the squamous layer (**b**)

Four to six pieces of biopsies are taken from the ATZ or cuff, pouch body, and afferent limb for surveillance purpose. Deep or tunnel biopsy of the ATZ or cuff is recommended in patients with a preoperative diagnosis of CAN (Fig. 6.3). In addition, any abnormal or suspicious areas, such as polyps, strictures, and deep ulcers, should be biopsied.

Image-enhanced pouchoscopy, such as chromoendoscopy and narrow-band imaging, may help improve the accuracy of surveillance endoscopy (Fig. 6.1).

Histologic Features of Pouch Neoplasia

Histological findings range from no dysplasia, indefinite for dysplasia, LGD, HGD, to cancer [15]. Commonly reported microscopic features include architectural alterations resulting from repair in chronic pouchitis and cytological abnormalities, after eliminating the possibility of regenerative and inflammatory changes that may affect the mucosa in chronic pouchitis [16]. Figure 6.3 is depicting unremarkable anal transitional zone. Deep biopsy showed cancer underneath the squamous layer. Pouch adenocarcinoma often appears to be mucinous and poorly differentiated type. An immunohistochemical study found that the source of pouch cancer originates from colorectal source, similar to UC-associated adenocarcinoma, rather than small bowel source [17]. It is advisable to obtain a sufficient number of biopsy samples and to control the underlying mucosal inflammation to augment diagnostic accuracy. The pathology report for pouch surveillance biopsy should clearly state the presence or absence of dysplasia. It is advisable to have the diagnosis of pouch neoplasia confirmed by at least two expert gastrointestinal pathologists with a particular interest in IBD.

Natural History of Pouch Neoplasia

ATZ or cuff is the most common site of development of pouch neoplasia [11]. LGD is the most commonly reported form of pouch neoplasia. Natural course, clinical significance, and management of LGD are yet to be defined. LGD has been reported to be able to regress; however, the risk for developing pouch cancer might have been higher if all LGD had progressed into HGD or cancer [7, 11]. Our previous study identified 44 patients with LGD, HGD, or adenocarcinoma in IPAA. Of the 22 patients with an initial diagnosis of pouch LGD, 6 had persistence or progression after a median follow-up of 9.5 years. Of the 12 patients with pouch HGD, 5 had a history of synchronous pouch LGD. Pouch HGD either persisted or progressed in three patients after the initial management, in a median time interval of 5.4 years. Of the 14 patients with pouch adenocarcinoma, 12 had a history of or synchronous dysplasia. After a median follow-up of 2.1 years, six patients with pouch cancer died [13]. The overall prognosis of pouch adenocarcinoma seems to be poor.

The histopathological term indefinite for dysplasia (IND) has been used to define a spectrum of atypical dysplastic features with concurrent inflammatory changes [18]. It was noted that the majority of patients with IND had concurrent mucosal inflammation on endoscopy and histology. It does not reach the threshold for an explicit diagnosis of true dysplasia by pathologists, and interobserver agreement in grading IND and LGD among GI pathologists has been poor. However, the natural history of IND seems to be benign, and progression to dysplasia or cancer is rare. On the other hand, the progression of IND or even chronic inflammation to neoplasia in UC patients is not unusual. Investigators have shown that 5-year progression rates to advanced neoplasia in patients with flat LGD and IND were 37% and 5%, respectively [19]. There is no consensus on the management of IND. Repeat pouchoscopy and image-enhanced endoscopy with extensive biopsy, along with an adequate control of concurrent inflammation, are recommended.

Endoscopy Surveillance for Pouch Neoplasia

There are no published guidelines or consensus for endoscopy surveillance for pouch neoplasia between professional societies. The British Society of Gastroenterology suggests an annual pouch endoscopy for high-risk patients such as those with previous rectal dysplasia, dysplasia or cancer at the time of pouch surgery, PSC, or type C mucosa of the pouch, persistent atrophy, and severe inflammation [20]. Surveillance is recommended every 5 years in all others. In our recent survey study, more than half of the physicians (55%) preferred that pouchoscopy should be performed every 2–3 years solely for the surveillance of pouch neoplasia. An annual surveillance pouchoscopy was favored by 23% of the physicians surveyed, and 18% chose an individualized plan. Only 2% of the physicians preferred a 5-year surveillance protocol [21].

Since the natural history of pouch neoplasia is poorly defined and the prognosis of pouch cancer is poor, we recommend a more aggressive approach. A standard surveillance protocol, taking into account the individual risk factors, should be considered instead.

We recommend that surveillance pouchoscopy and biopsy every 1–3 years be performed, beginning 10 years after the initial diagnosis of UC in patients without risk factors. In high-risk patients, including those with UC diagnosis for more than 10 years, chronic pouchitis or cuffitis, type C mucosa, marked inflammation in the lamina propria along with villous atrophy, family history of CRC in a first-degree relative, or PSC, pouchoscopy and biopsy should be performed every 1 to 3 years. In patients with preoperative neoplasia of the colon and/or rectum, pouchoscopy and biopsy should be done annually, with focus on the cuff or ATZ (Fig. 6.4) [14, 22, 23].

It may be reasonable to biopsy patients with LGD at intervals of 3–6 months, even after the lesion has been endoscopically removed.

Treatment of Pouch Neoplasia

Polypectomy or endoscopic mucosal resection (EMR) with close endoscopic surveillance may be attempted for patients with isolated polypoid LGD. Well-defined, small (<1–2 cm) endoscopically liftable unifocal LGD may be treated with EMR or endoscopic submucosal dissection (ESD). Ideally, the lesion should be removed en bloc. In addition, extensive biopsy should be taken from adjacent mucosa. Unifocal slightly raised LGD should undergo pouchoscopy with biopsy, with or without prior

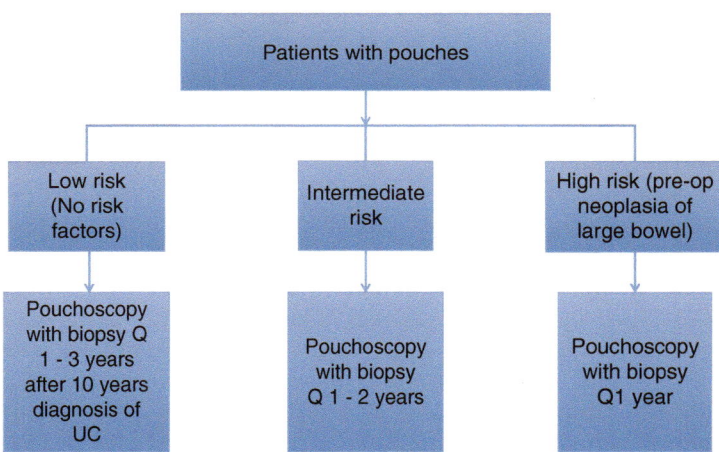

Fig. 6.4 Surveillance algorithm for pouch neoplasia

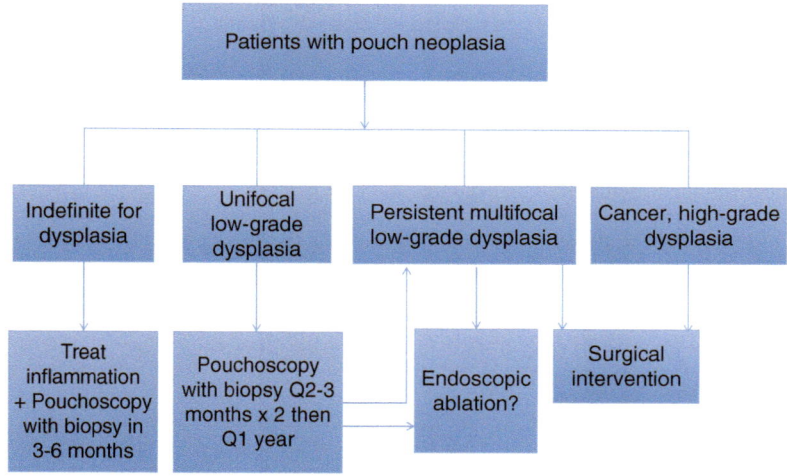

Fig. 6.5 Management algorithm for pouch neoplasia

endoscopic ablation, every 2–3 months × 2 and then every year if dysplasia is not detected in the subsequent biopsies [14].

Surgical invention is typically required for patients with pouch cancer, HGD, persistent, multifocal LGD, or flat LGD or HGD [15]. Some investigators recommended surgical mucosectomy and pouch advancement procedure while others suggested pouch excision for pouch-associated HGD [11, 24, 25]. Surgical interventions, such as completion proctectomy, may be required, especially for patients with risk factors for neoplastic progression or recurrence, such as preoperative diagnosis of colorectal neoplasia or family history of CRC [11]. Pouch excision is the appropriate choice of therapy should pouch HGD persist [11]. Because pouch neoplasia appears to have a poor prognosis, early detection of dysplasia with pouchoscopy surveillance may offer the best approach (Fig. 6.5) [15].

Summary

Pouch neoplasia is infrequent but potentially lethal adverse sequelae in patients with underlying IBD following IPAA. Proper follow-up is recommended to develop an optimal surveillance strategy in patients with suspected pouch neoplasia. A majority of pouch adenocarcinoma cases seem to follow a carcinogenic pathway similar to that of UC-associated cancer [14]. An algorithm for surveillance and management is proposed (Figs. 6.4 and 6.5).

Disclosure The authors declared no financial conflict of interest.

References

1. Delaney CP, Fazio VW, Remzi FH, et al. Prospective, age-related analysis of surgical results, functional outcome, and quality of life after ileal pouch-anal anastomosis. Ann Surg. 2003;238:221–8.
2. Fazio VW, Kiran RP, Remzi FH, et al. Ileal pouch anal anastomosis: analysis of outcome and quality of life in 3707 patients. Ann Surg. 2013;257:679–85.
3. Delaney CP, Remzi FH, Gramlich T, et al. Equivalent function, quality of life and pouch survival rates after ileal pouch-anal anastomosis for indeterminate and ulcerative colitis. Ann Surg. 2002;236:43–8.
4. Scarpa M, van Koperen PJ, Ubbink DT, et al. Systematic review of dysplasia after restorative proctocolectomy for ulcerative colitis. Br J Surg. 2007;94:534–45.
5. O'Riordain MG, Fazio VW, Lavery IC, et al. Incidence and natural history of dysplasia of the anal transitional zone after ileal pouch-anal anastomosis: results of a five-year to ten-year follow-up. Dis Colon Rectum. 2000;43:1660–5.
6. Shepherd NA, Jass JR, Duval I, et al. Restorative proctocolectomy with ileal reservoir: pathological and histochemical study of mucosal biopsy specimens. J Clin Pathol. 1987;40:601–7.
7. Ziv Y, Fazio VW, Sirimarco MT, et al. Incidence, risk factors, and treatment of dysplasia in the anal transitional zone after ileal pouch-anal anastomosis. Dis Colon Rectum. 1994;37:1281–5.
8. Banasiewicz T, Marciniak R, Paszkowski J, et al. Pouchitis may increase the risk of dysplasia after restorative proctocolectomy in patients with ulcerative colitis. Color Dis. 2012;14:92–7.
9. Chambers WM, Mc CMNJ. Should ileal pouch-anal anastomosis include mucosectomy? Color Dis. 2007;9:384–92.
10. Kariv R, Remzi FH, Lian L, et al. Preoperative colorectal neoplasia increases risk for pouch neoplasia in patients with restorative proctocolectomy. Gastroenterology. 2010;139:806–12.
11. Derikx LA, Kievit W, Drenth JP, et al. Prior colorectal neoplasia is associated with increased risk of ileoanal pouch neoplasia in patients with inflammatory bowel disease. Gastroenterology. 2014;146:119–28.
12. Remzi FH, Fazio VW, Delaney CP, et al. Dysplasia of the anal transitional zone after ileal pouch-anal anastomosis: results of prospective evaluation after a minimum of ten years. Dis Colon Rectum. 2003;46:6–13.
13. Wu XR, Remzi FH, Liu XL, et al. Disease course and management strategy of pouch neoplasia in patients with underlying inflammatory bowel diseases. Inflamm Bowel Dis. 2014;20:2073–82.
14. Liu ZX, Kiran RP, Bennett AE, et al. Diagnosis and management of dysplasia and cancer of the ileal pouch in patients with underlying inflammatory bowel disease. Cancer. 2011;117:3081–92.
15. Schaus BJ, Fazio VW, Remzi FH, et al. Clinical features of ileal pouch polyps in patients with underlying ulcerative colitis. Dis Colon Rectum. 2007;50:832–8.
16. Gonzalo DH, Collinsworth AL, Liu X. Common inflammatory disorders and neoplasia of the ileal pouch: a review of histopathology. Gastroenterology Res. 2016;9:29–38.
17. Jiang W, Shadrach B, Carver P, Goldblum JR, Shen B, Liu X. Histomorphologic and molecular features of pouch and peripouch adenocarcinoma: a comparison with ulcerative colitis-associated adenocarcinoma. Am J Surg Pathol. 2012;36:1385–94.
18. Liu ZX, Liu XL, Patil DT, et al. Clinical significance of indefinite for dysplasia on pouch biopsy in patients with underlying inflammatory bowel disease. J Gastrointest Surg. 2012;16:562–71.
19. Van Schaik FD, Ten Kate FJ, Offerhaus GJ, et al. Misclassification of dysplasia in patients with inflammatory bowel disease: consequences for progression rates to advanced neoplasia. Inflamm Bowel Dis. 2011;17:1108–16.
20. Eaden JA, Mayberry JF, British Society for Gastroenterology, Association of Coloproctology for Great Britain and Ireland. Guidelines for screening and surveillance of asymptomatic colorectal cancer in patients with inflammatory bowel disease. Gut. 2002;5:10.

21. Gu J, Remzi FH, Lian L, et al. Practice pattern of ileal pouch surveillance in academic medical centers in the United States. Gastroenterol Rep. 2016;4:119–24.
22. Gadacz TR, McFadden DW, Gabrielson EW, et al. Adenocarcinoma of the ileostomy: the latent risk of cancer after colectomy for ulcerative colitis and familial polyposis. Surgery. 1990;107:698.
23. Smart PJ, Sastry S, Wells S. Primary mucinous adenocarcinoma developing in an ileostomy stoma. Gut. 1988;29:1607.
24. Coull DB, Lee FD, Henderson AP, et al. Risk of dysplasia in the columnar cuff after stapled restorative proctocolectomy. Br J Surg. 2003;90:72.
25. Heuschen UA, Heuschen G, Autschbach F, et al. Adenocarcinoma in the ileal pouch: late risk of cancer after restorative proctocolectomy. Int J Color Dis. 2001;16:126–30.

Chapter 7
Other Cancers: Small-Bowel Cancers, Cholangiocarcinoma, Urinary Tract, and Anal Cancer Risk and Screening in Inflammatory Bowel Disease

Fernanda Dal Bello and Alan C. Moss

Introduction

It has long been recognized that patients with long-standing inflammatory bowel disease (IBD) are at increased risk for the development of various neoplasms, particularly colorectal cancer (CRC), but also cervical cancer and skin cancer, among others. Chronic inflammation in the colon and biliary tree can induce a broad array of neoplastic pathways in affected organs [1]. However, in other organs that do not exhibit chronic inflammation, long-term exposure to immunosuppressive therapies is the risk factor most associated with cancer development. Agents such as thiopurines and anti-TNFs can introduce oncogenic viral infections, acquired genetic mutations, or susceptibility to UVA damage that can trigger malignant transformation in cells in the skin, lymphatic system, and cervix among others [2]. Although these cancers remain rare in IBD patients, an understanding of their risk factors and clinical presentation is important for prevention strategies and early detection. For this chapter, we have focused on small intestinal, biliary, urinary, and anal cancers. The main characteristics of the cancer screening are in Table 7.1.

F. D. Bello · A. C. Moss (✉)
Division of Gastroenterology, Center for Inflammatory Bowel Disease, Beth Israel Deaconess
Medical Center, Boston, MA, USA
e-mail: amoss@bidmc.harvard.edu

© Springer Nature Switzerland AG 2019
J. D. Feuerstein, A. S. Cheifetz (eds.), *Cancer Screening in Inflammatory Bowel Disease*, https://doi.org/10.1007/978-3-030-15301-4_7

Table 7.1 Risk factors and screening recommendations

	Risk factors	Screening and recommendations
Small-bowel cancer (adenocarcinoma is the most frequent subtype)	Chronic inflammation Long disease duration Distal jejunal/ileal localization Strictures and fistulae	No specific recommendations
Cholangiocarcinoma	*PSC* Smoking Alcohol Duration of IBD Previous CRC Previous dysplasia HLA-DR4/DQ8 Dominant stenosis	In patients with PSC Annual CA 19-9 US or MRI every 6–12 months
Urinary tract cancer	Age (≥65 years) Male gender Use of thiopurines	No specific recommendations
Anal cancer	HPV infection Chronic inflammation Perianal disease	Routine prophylactic HPV vaccination Annual perianal clinical examination

UC ulcerative colitis, *CD* Crohn's disease, *PSC* primary sclerosing cholangitis, *US* ultrasound, *MRI* magnetic resonance, *HPV* human papillomavirus

Small-Bowel Cancer

Epidemiology

Small-bowel cancer is uncommon, accounting for approximately 2% of all neoplasms of the gastrointestinal tract [3, 4]. Adenocarcinoma is the most frequent subtype, but sarcomas, lymphomas, and carcinoids have all been identified in patients with ileal CD. The estimated incidence of small intestinal adenocarcinoma in CD patients is 0.3/1000 patient-years [5, 6, 7]. A population-based study from Denmark generated a relative risk of small-bowel adenocarcinoma of 60 in patients with CD, compared to the background population [8]. Diagnosis typically occurs late in the disease course, with a mean duration of 8 years of established disease before diagnosis of small intestinal adenocarcinoma [9]. With an overall prevalence in the Crohn's disease population of ~1%, this cancer still remains an infrequent finding in absolute terms [10].

Risk Factors/Pathogenesis

Patients with chronic inflammation in their small bowel are at increased risk for the development of neoplasms in this location. In patients with CD, long disease duration, distal jejunal/ileal localization, and complications such as strictures and fistulae are disease factors consistently associated with the development of small-bowel cancer [11]. Patient factors that have also been linked to an increased risk include young age at diagnosis, male gender, and smoking. It is likely that many of the risk factors identified are surrogate markers for complicated ileal disease. The role of medication exposure is inconsistent, as are occupational risk factors [12, 13]. A case-control study published in 2008 showed that prior resection of the small intestine and the use of aminosalicylates for a period of more than 2 years significantly decreased the incidence of adenocarcinoma in the small intestine [14].

Screening Methods and Recommendations

Small intestinal cancers are infrequent, usually diagnosed only at the time of intestinal resection, and often as incidental findings [15]. As a consequence, identification of early-stage lesions is a challenge and, given their rarity, would not warrant routine screening in the CD population. No professional bodies currently recommend routine screening for small-bowel cancer, even in high-risk populations.

Symptomatic patients with new stenosis during clinical remission or stenosis refractory to therapy should be investigated [7]. In patients with CD, differentiating a benign inflammatory stricture from an early-stage small-bowel tumor can be difficult, so often the diagnosis is made only by the pathologist on examination of resected segments [5]. On CT or MRI, adenocarcinoma may present as a sacculated loop with asymmetrical thickening or as a short segment of stenosis mimicking benign fibrostenosis [14, 16]. Alternative diagnostic approaches in symptomatic patients include ileocolonoscopy, PET scans, and capsule endoscopy. Capsule endoscopy has displayed 83% sensitivity for tumor detection with a negative predictive value of 97%, but does not allow biopsy collection [7].

Cholangiocarcinoma

Epidemiology

Cholangiocarcinoma (CC) is the second commonest primary liver tumor worldwide, after hepatocellular carcinoma (HCC). CC develops in cholangiocytes, with malignant transformation triggered by infection, inflammation, and cholestasis. Incidence and mortality rates for intrahepatic CC have risen steeply and steadily across the world over the past few decades with concomitant falls in extrahepatic CC rates [17]. Primary sclerosing cholangitis (PSC) is the main known risk factor, which may occur in the presence or absence of IBD. It is estimated that the risk of developing cholangiocarcinoma in patients with PSC is 0.5–1.5% per year, with a lifetime prevalence of 5–20% [18, 19].

Risk Factors/Pathogenesis

Patients with IBD, especially with UC, are at higher risk for developing cholangio-carcinoma than the general population, and this increase is mainly caused by the association of this cancer with PSC. Primary sclerosing cholangitis is the common-est known predisposing factor in the Western world; the 10-year cumulative risk is around 8% [19]. In addition to cholangiocarcinoma (CC), an increased frequency of gallbladder carcinoma (GBC), hepatocellular carcinoma (HCC), and colorectal car-cinoma (CRC) is also observed in patients with PSC. Studies report that the risk of intrahepatic CC is increased in patients with UC, but not in CD patients [20]. The severity of liver disease does not appear to be a significant risk factor. Smoking, alcohol, duration of IBD, previous CRC/dysplasia and the HLA-DR4, and DQ8 haplotype are reported risk factors for CC in patients with PSC [21]. The presence of dominant stenosis/strictures (defined as a stricture less than 1.5 mm diameter in the common bile duct or less than 1 mm in the left or right main hepatic ducts) when accompanied with IBD also seems to be associated with an increased risk of biliary cancer [22]. Evaluation of these strictures is important, as among patients with chol-angiocarcinoma, almost half of the malignancies were diagnosed within the first 4 months after initial diagnosis of PSC [19]. In longitudinal studies of small duct PSC, biliary cancer has not been reported unless there is progression to large duct PSC [23]. Thus, although all IBD patients with PSC are at increased risk of CC, there are individual factors that stratify risk within PSC groups.

Screening Methods and Recommendations

Most experts agree that early detection of CC in PSC may identify cases amenable to curative surgery and avoid inappropriate liver transplantation [24, 25]. Screening for cholangiocarcinoma with regular (every 6–12 months) cross-sectional imaging with ultrasound or MRI, and serial CA 19-9 measures, is recommended by the American College of Gastroenterology, but this is based on expert opinion only [26]. More recent expert opinions have suggested only annual MRI and CA 19-9 [27]. No studies have documented that this approach leads to a reduction in mortal-ity from CC in patients with PSC, so the benefits and cost-effectiveness of this strategy have not been confirmed.

There are limitations to this approach. A CA19-9 cutoff of 129 U/mL has a reported sensitivity and specificity of 79% and 99% (respectively) for CCA detec-tion, and a threshold of 100 U/mL yielded a similar diagnostic performance. However, only advanced cases of CCA were detected by either cutoff [28]. Complicating use of this biomarker, 7% of the population are unable to produce CA19-9, and one third of PSC patients with a CA 19-9 greater than 129 U/mL do not have underlying CCA [29]. Consequently, ACG guidelines on management of focal liver lesions do not support routine screening for CCA in patients with under-lying PSC, despite the increased incidence of CCA in this population [30]. Both European Crohn's and Colitis Organization (ECCO) and the British Society of

Gastroenterology (BSG) guidelines do not recommend routine screening for chol-angiocarcinoma in IBD patients, but emphasize the importance of clinical manage-ment of the risk of biliary cancer in patients with PSC.

Urinary Tract Cancer

Epidemiology and Risk Factors

The risk of urinary tract cancers, including kidney and bladder cancers, are increased in patients with IBD and those receiving immunosuppressive therapy. Overall, IBD patients have an increased risk of cancer of the urinary bladder (SIR 2.03) [31]. Incidence rates for urinary tract malignancy are threefold higher in IBD patients ≥65 years of age when compared with cancer IRs in the SEER database for the same age group (IR 0.37/100 PY vs. 0.12/100 PY), independent of immunomodula-tor or biologic use [32]. The reasons for this increased risk are uncertain, although differences in smoking rates and immunosuppression have been postulated. Once diagnosed, IBD patients have a significantly lower age at renal cell cancer diagno-sis, are at earlier stage at diagnosis, and are more likely to undergo surgical treat-ment compared to the general population. This translated into better survival, independent of immunosuppression in one study [33].

Risk factors for urinary cancer in IBD patients include the use of thiopurines (HR 2.8), male gender (HR 3.9), and increasing age (HR after 65 years 13.3) [34]. Specifically, for renal cell cancer, pancolitis (OR 1.8–2.5), penetrating Crohn's dis-ease (OR 2.8), and IBD-related surgery were also identified as independent risk factors [33].

Screening Methods and Recommendations

There are no specific recommendations in the current guidelines for screening for urinary tract neoplasia in IBD patients, given their rarity and lack of suitable screen-ing tests for early cancers. In older male patients, the highest risk group, incidental lesions on CT/MRI or urinary symptoms should be promptly investigated.

Anal Cancer

Epidemiology

Patients with IBD are at risk of developing both anal squamous cell carcinoma (SCC) and anal adenocarcinoma. These have been attributed to human papilloma virus (HPV) infection (squamous) and chronic inflammation (squamous and adenocarcinoma) of the anal mucosa [35]. In a large cohort study in France of 2911 patients with perianal Crohn's disease, 2 patients were diagnosed with anal SCC and 3 patients with perianal fistula-related anal adenocarcinoma during follow-up. This translated to incidence rates of 0.26 per 1000 patient-years for anal squamous-cell carcinoma and 0.38 per 1000 patient-years for perianal fistula-related adenocarcinoma [36]. For patients with UC, or no perianal disease, the incidence rate for SCC was even lower, 0.08 per 1000 patient-years. Of note, the risk of rectal adenocarcinoma was fivefold higher in patients with perianal Crohn's disease than those without perianal disease in this study.

Anal SCC in IBD has a poor prognosis, with a 37% 5-year survival rate, in contrast to 60% 5-year survival in the general population [37]. The prognosis of perianal fistula-associated cancers is also poor, with a 4-year survival rate ranging among series from 30% to 60% [34]. In both conditions, delay in diagnosis due to nonspecific symptoms, and challenges in acquiring malignant cells during sampling of fistula tracts, is thought to explain these poorer outcomes.

Risk Factors/Pathogenesis

HPV infection and chronic inflammation are the two established risk factors for anal cancer in patients with IBD. It is known that HPV is a risk factor for SCC, and a majority of IBD patients (89%) had anal human papillomavirus when screened in one small study [38]. Whether chronic immunosuppression exposure plays a role in this risk is unclear. Although studies of HPV and cervical dysplasia have been linked to thiopurines, the two published studies on anal SCC have not been associated with thiopurines [36, 39]. For adenocarcinomas, chronic inflammation related to perianal disease was the sole factor significantly associated with a higher risk of anal cancer (odds ratio 11) in one study in patients with Crohn's disease [36].

Screening Methods and Recommendations

Given the association between HPV and SCC, routine prophylactic HPV vaccination is recommended for both females and males according to national guidelines [40]. Apart from this, the risk of non-fistula-related SCC in patients with IBD is low, and similar to the general population, therefore does not justify an anal cancer screening program in patients with IBD without other risk factors (HIV infection, urogenital condyloma).

In contrast, the higher incidence of rectal cancer and anal adenocarcinoma in patients with perianal CD warrants further consideration. No guidelines for surveillance intervals or modalities have been established to date, although the practice has been recommended [35]. In the absence of such guidelines, we recommend annual examination of the perineum to identify changes in morphology or findings over time. In particular, any patient with new or change in anal symptoms should have a perianal clinical examination, including digital rectal examination, followed by anoscopy and biopsies, and/or MRI when malignancy is suspected. Unexplained pain should always raise the suspicion of anal cancer. Given the low yield or clinical examination and imaging, there should be a low threshold for examination under anesthesia and biopsy/curettage of fistula tracts in this setting [41].

Conclusion

Patients with IBD are at a higher risk of cancer in extra-colonic locations. Although these cancers are rare, they are often diagnosed late in their course. Their low incidence, lack of suitable screening modalities, and lack of evidence of an impact of screening on mortality have not led to recommendations for universal screening in patients with IBD to date (except CC). However, clinicians should remain vigilant to new or altered symptoms attributable to these organs with this knowledge in mind.

References

1. Ullman TA, Itzkowitz SH. Intestinal inflammation and cancer. Gastroenterology. 2011;140(6):1807–16.
2. O'Donovan P, Perrett CM, Zhang X, et al. Azathioprine and UVA light generate mutagenic oxidative DNA damage. Science. 2005;309:1871–4.
3. DiSario JA, Burt RW, Vargas H, et al. Small bowel cancer: epidemiological and clinical characteristics from a population-based registry. Am J Gastroenterol. 1994;89:699–701.
4. Chow JS, Chen CC, Ahsan H, et al. A population-based study of the incidence of malignant small-bowel tumors: SEER 1973–1990. Int J Epidemiol. 1996;25:722–8.
5. Lichtenstein GR, Loftus EV, Isaacs KL, et al. ACG clinical guideline: management of Crohn's disease in adults. Am J Gastroenterol. 2018;113(4):481–517.
6. Annese V, Daperno M, Rutter MD, et al. European evidence based consensus for endoscopy in inflammatory bowel disease. J Crohns Colitis. 2013;7:982–1018.
7. ECCO Guideline. European evidence-based consensus: inflammatory bowel disease and malignancies. J Crohns Colitis. 2015.
8. Jess T, Winther KV, Munkholm P, Langholz E, Binder V. Intestinal and extra-intestinal cancer in Crohn's disease: follow-up of population-based cohort in Copenhagen County, Denmark. Aliment Pharmacol Ther. 2004.
9. Elriz K, Carrat F, Carbonnel F, et al. Incidence, presentation, and prognosis of small bowel adenocarcinoma in patients with small bowel Crohn's disease: a prospective observational study. Inflamm Bowel Dis. 2013.
10. Shaukat A, Virnig DJ, Howard D, Sitaraman SV, Liff JM, Lederle FA. Crohn's disease and small bowel adenocarcinoma: a population-based case-control study. Cancer Epidemiol Biomark Prev. 2011;20(6):1120–3.
11. Cahill C, Gordon PH, Petrucci A, Boutros M. Small bowel adenocarcinoma and Crohn's disease: any further ahead than 50 years ago?. World J Gastroenterol. 2014.
12. Lashner BA. Risk factors for small bowel cancer in Crohn's disease. Dig Dis Sci. 1992;37(8):1179–84.

13. Solem CA, Harmsen WS et al. Small intestinal adenocarcinoma in Crohn's disease: a case-control study. Inflamm Bowel Dis. 2004.
14. Piton G, Cosnes J, Monnet E, et al. Risk factors associated with small bowel adenocarcinoma in Crohn's disease: a case-control study. Am J Gastroenterol. 2008.
15. Dossett LA, White LM, Welch DC, et al. Small bowel adenocarcinoma complicating Crohn's disease: case series and review of the literature. Am Surg. 2007;73(11):1181–7.
16. Tirkes AT, Duerinckx AJ. Adenocarcinoma of the ileum in Crohn disease. Abdom Imaging. 2005.
17. Welzel TM, McGlynn KA, Hsing AW, et al. Impact of classification of hilar cholangiocarcinomas (Klatskin tumors) on the incidence of intra and extrahepatic cholangiocarcinoma in the United States. J Natl Cancer Inst. 2006.
18. Khaderi SA, Sussman NL. Screening for malignancy in primary sclerosing cholangitis (PSC). Curr Gastroenterol Rep. 2015;17(4):17.
19. Burak K, Angulo P, Pasha TM, et al. Incidence and risk factors for cholangiocarcinoma in primary sclerosing cholangitis. Am J Gastroenterol. 2004;99(3):523–6.
20. Welzel TM, Mellemkjaer L, Gloria G, et al. Risk factors for intrahepatic cholangiocarcinoma in a low-risk population: a nationwide case-control study. Int J Cancer. 2007.
21. Khan SA, Davidson BR, Goldin RD, et al. Guidelines for the diagnosis and treatment of cholangiocarcinoma: an update. Gut. 2012.
22. Rudolph G, Gotthardt D, Kloeters-Plachky P, Rost D, et al. In PSC with dominant bile duct stenosis, IBD is associated with an increase of carcinomas and reduced survival. J Hepatol. 2010;53(2):313–7.
23. Singal AK, Stanca CM, Clark V, Dixon L, et al. Natural history of small duct primary sclerosing cholangitis: a case series with review of the literature. Hepatol Int. 2011;5(3):808–13.
24. Chapman RW, Fevery J, Kalloo A, et al. AASLD practice guidelines: diagnosis and management of primary sclerosing cholangitis. Hepatology. 2010.
25. Beuers U, Boberg KM, Chapman RW, et al. EASL clinical practice guidelines: management of cholestatic liver diseases. J Hepatol. 2009.
26. Lindor KD, Kowdley KV, Harrison E. ACG clinical guideline: primary sclerosing cholangitis. Am J Gastroenterol. 2015;110:646–59.
27. Rizvi S, Eaton JE, Gores GJ. Primary sclerosing cholangitis as a premalignant biliary tract disease: surveillance and management. Clin Gastroenterol Hepatol. 2015.
28. Levy C, Lymp J, Angulo P, et al. The value of serum CA 19-9 in predicting cholangiocarcinomas in patients with primary sclerosing cholangitis. Dig Dis Sci. 2005;50(9):1734–40.
29. Sinakos E, Saenger AK, Keach J, Kim WR, Lindor KD. Many patients with primary sclerosing cholangitis and increased serum levels of carbohydrate antigen 19-9 do not have cholangiocarcinoma. Clin Gastroenterol Hepatol. 2011.
30. Marrero JA, Ahn J, Rajender RK. ACG clinical guideline: the diagnosis and management of focal liver lesions. Am J Gastroenterol. 2014.
31. Pedersen N, Duricova D, Elkjaer M, et al. Risk of extra-intestinal cancer in inflammatory bowel disease: meta-analysis of population-based cohort studies. Am J Gastroenterol. 2010.
32. Khan N, Vallarino C, Lissoos T, Darr U, Luo M. Risk of malignancy in a nationwide cohort of elderly inflammatory bowel disease patientes. Drugs Aging. 2017.
33. Derikx LA, Nissen LH, Drenth JP, et al. Better survival of renal cell carcinoma in patients with inflammatory bowel disease. Oncotarget. 2015;6(35):38336–47.
34. Bourrier A, Carrat F, Colombel JF, et al. Excess risk of urinary tract cancers in patients receiving thiopurines for inflammatory bowel disease: a prospective observational cohort study. Aliment Pharmacol Ther. 2016.
35. Wisniewski A, Flejou JF, Siproudhis L, et al. Anal neoplasia in inflammatory bowel disease: classification proposal, epidemiology, carcinogenesis, and risk management perspectives. J Crohns Colitis. 2017.
36. Beaugerie L, Carrat F, Nahon S, et al. High risk of anal and rectal cancer in patients with anal and/or perianal Crohn's disease. Clin Gastroenterol Hepatol. 2018.

37. Slesser AA, Bhangu A, Bower M, Goldin R, Tekkis PP. A systematic review of anal squamous cell carcinoma in inflammatory bowel disease. Surg Oncol. 2013.
38. Cranston RD, Regueiro M, Hashash J, et al. A pilot study of the prevalence of anal human papillomavirus and dysplasia in a cohort of patients with IBD. Dis Colon Rectum. 2017.
39. Shah SB, Pickham D, Araya H, et al. Prevalence of anal dysplasia in patients with inflammatory bowel disease. Clin Gastroenterol Hepatol. 2015;13:1955–61.
40. Rahier JF, Magro F, Abreu C, et al. Second European evidence-based consensus on the prevention, diagnosis and management of opportunist infections in inflammatory bowel disease. J Crohns Colitis. 2014.
41. Devon KM, Brown CJ, Burnstein M, et al. Cancer of the anus complicating perianal Crohn's disease. Dis Colon Rectum. 2009;52:211–6.

Chapter 8
Cancer Risks and Screening with Current and Emerging Drug Therapies in Inflammatory Bowel Diseases

Helen Lee, Yecheskel Schneider, and Gary R. Lichtenstein

What's the Risk of Lymphomas in the General Population?

The two main categories of lymphomas, cancers of the immune system, are non-Hodgkin's lymphoma (NHL) and Hodgkin's lymphoma (HL). HL arises from mature B cells, while NHL can come from mature B, T, and/or NK cells [1, 2]. NHL, the seventh most common cancer in the USA, occurs more frequently than HL, but together they account for about 5% of new cancers diagnosed in the USA annually [1–3]. The National Cancer Institute's Surveillance, Epidemiology, and End Results (SEER) Program estimates that there will be 74,680 new cases of NHL in the USA in 2018, accounting for 4.3% of all new cancers, and 19,910 (3.3%) estimated deaths from all cancers (see Table 8.1) [3]. SEER estimates that there will be 8500 new cases of HL diagnosed in the USA in 2018 accounting for 0.5% of new

Helen Lee and Yecheskel Schneider contributed equally to the work and are co-first authors.

H. Lee · Y. Schneider
Division of Gastroenterology, Department of Medicine, Hospital of the University of Pennsylvania, Philadelphia, PA, USA

University of Pennsylvania School of Medicine, Philadelphia, PA, USA
e-mail: Helen.Lee2@uphs.upenn.edu; Yecheskel.Schneider@pennmedicine.upenn.edu

G. R. Lichtenstein (✉)
Division of Gastroenterology, Department of Medicine, Hospital of the University of Pennsylvania, Philadelphia, PA, USA

University of Pennsylvania School of Medicine, Philadelphia, PA, USA

Center for Inflammatory Bowel Diseases, The Raymond and Ruth Perelman School of Medicine of the University of Pennsylvania, Philadelphia, PA, USA

Gastroenterology Division, Department of Internal Medicine, Perelman Center for Advanced Medicine, Philadelphia, PA, USA
e-mail: Gary.lichtenstein@uphs.upenn.edu

© Springer Nature Switzerland AG 2019   95
J. D. Feuerstein, A. S. Cheifetz (eds.), *Cancer Screening in Inflammatory Bowel Disease*, https://doi.org/10.1007/978-3-030-15301-4_8

Table 8.1 Epidemiology of NHL and HL [3]

	NHL	HL
Prevalence compared to other types of cancer in the USA	#7	#26
Estimated new cases in 2018 (%)	74,680 (4.3)	8500 (0.5)
Estimated deaths in 2018 (%)	19, 910 (3.3)	1, 020 (0.2)
Lifetime risk (%)	2.1	0.2
New cases per 100,000 people per year (between 2011 and 2015)	19.4	2.5
New deaths per 100,000 people per year (between 2011 and 2015)	5.7	0.3

Source: Surveillance, Epidemiology, and End Results (SEER) Program. https://seer.cancer.gov/

cancers and 1050 estimated deaths from HL or 0.2% of all cancer deaths [3]. Some risk factors for NHL include older age (median age of diagnosis is 67 years old), race (Caucasian >black), gender (slight predominance in males over females), inherited or acquired immunocompromised status (patients with human immunodeficiency virus, organ transplant, or autoimmune disorder or on immunosuppressants), and infections (Epstein-Barr virus, HTLV-1, HIV, *Helicobacter pylori*, hepatitis C, human herpesvirus 8) [1, 3]. The estimated lifetime risk for developing NHL is 2.1% [3]. Some risk factors for HL include race (Caucasian, black), age (young adults between 20 and 34 years old; median age of diagnosis is 39-SEER), gender (males over females), and presence of an inherited or acquired immunocompromised condition similar to the risk factors for NHL [2–4]. The estimated lifetime risk for developing HL is 0.2% [3].

Does Having IBD Increase a Patient's Risk for Lymphoma?

Although some earlier observational studies that were conducted largely at referral centers reported there was an associated increased risk for lymphoma among patients with IBD, several population-based studies later revealed that the risk of lymphomas for IBD patients who are not on immunosuppressive therapies is similar to the general population [5–16]. In 2000, Loftus et al. published the results of a population-based cohort study on IBD patients diagnosed between 1940 and 1993 in Olmsted County, Minnesota, before the advent of immunomodulators and biologic therapies to assess whether those patients with IBD had a higher risk for NHL [17]. They found that the absolute risk was negligible at 0.01% per person-year [17]. A subsequent retrospective cohort study by Lewis et al. in 2001 using the General Practice Research Database (GPRD) from the UK reached a similar conclusion [18]. The GPRD was felt to be representative of the country's entire population [18]. The study included over 16,000 patients with IBD and compared them to greater than 60,000 matched control patients without IBD to determine if there was a greater incidence of NHL or HL in patients with IBD [18]. They found that the relative risk (RR) of lymphoma (either NHL or HL) in IBD patients compared to matched controls was not statistically significant with RR of 1.2 and 95% confidence interval (CI) of 0.7–2.1 [18]. Another large population-based study from Sweden that included more than 47,000 patients with IBD with prospectively collected data found that the standardized incidence ratio of lymphomas was 0.8 with 95% CI of 0.5–1.3 in patients with UC and 1.3 with 95% CI of 0.8–2.0 in patients with Crohn's [19].

There were two population-based studies that showed different conclusions. One from Manitoba, Canada, found that there is an increased risk of lymphoma in male Crohn's patients, while another study from Florence, Italy, noted an increased risk of HL in patients with ulcerative colitis [20, 21]. However, these conflicting findings were not confirmed by other population-based studies.

Based on the large amount of evidence amassed from several population-based studies conducted in the past two decades, having IBD likely confers an insignificant to no increased risk for lymphoproliferative diseases [22–25].

What's the Risk of Skin Cancers in the General Population?

Melanomas and nonmelanoma skin cancers (NMSC) are the two main categories of cancer of the skin. Melanoma, cancer of melanocytes, is the fifth most common type of cancer in the USA [3]. According to SEER, the estimated number of new melanoma cases in 2018 is 91,270 which accounts for 5.3% of all cancers [3]. A similar estimated number of new cases of melanoma-in-situ will be diagnosed (87,290) in 2018 [26]. The estimated number of deaths from melanoma in 2018 is 9320 or 1.5% of all cancer deaths [3]. 2.3% of population will be diagnosed with melanoma in their lifetime [3]. Risk factors for melanomas include male gender, fair complexion, older age, cumulative exposure to ultraviolet light, history of sunburns, family or personal history of melanomas, presence of multiple atypical large nevi, congenital melanocytic nevi, certain geographic locations (highest incidence in New Zealand and Australia where the ozone layer is the thinnest), presence of mutation or deletion of cyclin-dependent kinase inhibitor 2A (CDKN2A), and/or presence of a variant melanocortin-1 receptor (MC1R) that produces melanins that are not sun-protective [3, 27, 28].

Although NMSC is the most commonly occurring cancer, its exact incidence in the USA is not clear as this information is not currently routinely collected and recorded in cancer registries [28]. There is an estimated annual incidence of at least 1.5–2 million cases of NMSC in the USA though that is likely an underestimate. One study estimated the total number of NMSC in the USA in 2012 to be greater than five million after analyzing administrative data from Centers for Medicare & Medicaid Services Physicians Claims database and population-based data from National Ambulatory Medical Care Survey database [28, 29]. NMSC encompasses both basal cell skin cancers and squamous cell skin cancers [28]. The majority of NMSC are basal cell skin cancers (70–80%), while squamous cell skin cancers comprise much of the remaining NMSC [28]. It is estimated that 20% of Americans will develop a skin cancer in their lifetime [30, 31]. Risk factors for developing NMSC are similar to melanomas, including cumulative and childhood ultraviolet light exposure, geographic location (relative to ozone layer thickness), older age, male gender, fair complexion, presence of certain skin conditions (xeroderma pigmentosum, epidermodysplasia verruciformis, nevoid basal cell cancer syndrome), exposures to ionizing radiation, immunosuppressed status, human papillomavirus infection, and chemical carcinogens like tobacco and arsenic [28, 31, 32].

Does Having IBD Increase a Patient's Risk for Skin Cancers?

IBD appears to be a risk factor for melanomas independent of immunomodulator (IMM) and biologic therapy exposure. A meta-analysis of 12 studies which included a total of 172,837 patients and 179 cases of melanoma diagnosed between 1940 and 2009 by Singh et al. in 2014 found that there is a 37% increased risk of melanoma in patients with Crohn's disease and ulcerative colitis over the general population [33]. The increased risk was seen in cohort studies predating the use of immunomodulators and anti-tumor necrosis factor alpha therapy as well as in subgroup analysis where hospital-based studies were excluded leaving only population-based cohorts [33]. Extensive disease was noted to be a possible risk factor for melanoma among patients with IBD [34].

Patients with IBD are not likely to be at increased risk for NMSC over the general population if they have not had exposure to immunomodulators or biologic therapies [35]. Although there were few cohort studies that noted an association between IBD and NMSC, they either did not account for the confounder of exposure to IMM like thiopurines or increased healthcare utilization [9, 35–39]. One study did note that there may be an increased risk for basal cell skin cancer in certain group of IBD patients; males younger than age 50 with Crohn's disease were found to have a threefold increase risk of NMSC compared to those without IBD [38].

The Risk of Lymphoproliferative Disorders After Exposure to Thiopurines and Anti-TNF Alpha Therapies

One of the greatest concerns when using immunomodulators or biologics for the treatment of inflammatory bowel disease, whether alone or in combination, is the concern regarding the risk of lymphoma. Although effective at inducing or maintaining remission, the risk of lymphoma may impose significant concern on both the patient and the physician when selecting a therapy. In particular, combination therapy with a thiopurine and an anti-TNF agent may carry a greater risk than when each individual agent is used alone. Much of the data we have examining the risk of lymphoma for individuals receiving therapy for their IBD relies on individual cohort studies and meta-analyses of these studies.

Thiopurines

A large nationwide cohort study from France, by Lemaitre et al., examined the risk of lymphoma for individuals on thiopurines and found that the risk of lymphoma was increased in those exposed to thiopurine monotherapy compared to those unexposed to thiopurine or anti-TNF agents, with an adjusted hazard ratio of 2.6 [40]. Another cohort study examining nationwide data in the USA over a 10-year period for individuals with ulcerative colitis treated with thiopurines found that patients on thiopurine had a fourfold increase in the risk of lymphoma while in therapy, compared to individuals not exposed, and this risk increased with ongoing use of the medication [41]. Additionally, a meta-analysis looking at the risk of lymphoma in individuals with IBD on thiopurines found an increased risk of lymphoma in those taking thiopurines, compared to those unexposed to medication. It found that the risk did not persist after discontinuation of therapy. Additionally, the risk was greatest in those over the age of 50 or men under the age of 35. Additionally, the meta-analysis found that the risk increased after one year of thiopurine use, but it was not increased when the duration of use was less than one year [42]. Thiopurines, either alone or in combination with anti-TNF therapy, may also be associated with the risk of developing Hepatosplenic T-cell lymphoma (HSTCL), a rare but aggressive lymphoma with a high risk of mortality. A systematic review of 36 reported cases of patients who developed HSTCL found that most patients were men, were younger than 35 years of age, and had received either thiopurine monotherapy or thiopurine combination therapy with an anti-TNF agent. Overall, the use of thiopurines does appear to be associated with a small but increased risk of lymphoma. This risk does appear to decrease overtime after discontinuation of the medication.

Anti-TNF Agents

The literature regarding the risk of anti-TNF therapy and the development of lymphoma has been conflicting. Data from the Crohn's Therapy, Resource, Evaluation, and Assessment Tool (TREAT™) Registry did not find an increased risk of lymphoma for individuals treated with infliximab therapy alone [43]. In addition, a large nationwide cohort study in Denmark found that exposure to an anti-TNF agent was not associated with an increased risk of lymphoma [44]. However, in the cohort study from Lemaitre et al., the risk of lymphoma for those who received anti-TNF therapy, compared to those who were unexposed to anti-TNF therapy or thiopurines, was increased, with an adjusted hazard ratio of 2.41 [40]. This risk was slightly lower for those who received anti-TNF monotherapy, as opposed to those who received thiopurine monotherapy. At this time, it is difficult to say whether anti-TNF therapy alone is associated with an increased risk of lymphoma; however, any such risk would likely be small and less than the risk of lymphoma when exposed to thiopurines.

Combination Therapy of a Thiopurine with an Anti-TNF

In the study by Lemaitre et al., the risk of lymphoma was greatest when exposed to combination therapy with a thiopurine and anti-TNF, with an adjusted hazard ratio of 6.11 [40]. Another study examining data in the USA from 1996 to 2009 and including 16,023 patients with IBD found that combination therapy of anti-TNF with thiopurine was associated with an increased risk [45]. A meta-analysis from 2010 examined the risk of lymphoma for individuals who had received an immuno-modulator and an anti-TNF agent for the treatment of Crohn's, including 26 studies in their analysis, with 8905 patients and 1178 patient-years of follow-up. The authors found that the use of combination therapy was associated with a small but increased risk of lymphoma, with a standardized incidence ratio of 3.23 [46]. Notably, combination therapy has also been seen in individuals who have developed HSTCL, as mentioned above in the thiopurine subsection. Combination therapy may be associated with an increased risk of lymphoma, greater than the risk of thio-purines or anti-TNF therapy alone.

Additional Therapies

Methotrexate

There are no adequately powered studies specifically examining the risk of lym-phoma in patients with inflammatory bowel disease receiving methotrexate. One study by Farrell et al. studied 782 patients with IBD, 238 of whom had received immunosuppressive therapy. Two of four patients who developed lymphoma had previously received methotrexate, either alone or in combination with cyclosporine [47]. However, given the limited data regarding the risk of lymphoma for individu-als on methotrexate, it is difficult to draw a conclusion regarding the risk based on this one study.

Tofacitinib

Tofacitinib, a small molecule JAK-kinase inhibitor, approved by the Food and Drug Administration for UC and for rheumatoid arthritis, has limited data evaluating the risk of malignancy for patients with IBD. Data pooled from studies evaluating tofacitinib for individuals with rheumatoid arthritis and did not show an increased risk of lymphoma for those on therapy when compared to standardized incidence ratios from the Surveillance, Epidemiology and End Results data [48]. In the randomized controlled trial evaluating tofacitinib for the treatment of UC, there was one reported lymphoma [49, 50]. Data examining the risk of lymphoma for individuals with rheumatoid arthritis on Tofacitinib have found the rate of lymphoma to be within the expected range of patients with moderate-to-severe rheumatoid arthritis [48]. Additional studies are needed in the future to better evaluate the risk of lymphoma for individuals with IBD who are receiving this medication.

Ustekinumab

Ustekinumab which is a monoclonal antibody directed against the p40 component of the interleukins 12 and 23 is currently approved for the treatment of Crohn's disease. Data focusing on the lymphoma risk is limited to randomized controlled studies evaluating the efficacy of the medication for the treatment of Crohn's disease, which have not shown an increased risk of lymphoma [51]. To date, there are no large cohort studies in patients with IBD which have evaluated the risk of lymphoma for individuals receiving this therapy.

Vedolizumab

Vedolizumab is a selective anti-integrin, which targets alpha4-beta7 and is approved for both UC and Crohn's disease. A large prospective cohort study evaluating the safety of vedolizumab for one year of use in 294 patients did not reveal any incident lymphomas [52]. A systematic review including 2830 patients exposed to vedolizumab also did not reveal an increased risk of lymphoma [53].

The Risk of Skin Cancer After Exposure to Thiopurines and Anti-TNF Alpha Therapies: Discordant Results

Anti-TNF Alpha Therapies

Melanoma

There were a few retrospective studies that seem to indicate that use of anti-TNF alpha therapies is linked to an increase risk for developing melanomas [39, 54]. In their 2012 retrospective study, Long and her colleagues analyzed data from an insurance claims database and showed that there was an increased incidence of melanoma (IRR 1.29 with 95% CI 1.09–1.53) in IBD patients who used biologics, especially those with Crohn's disease (IRR 1.45 with 95% CI 1.13–1.85, adjusted HR 1.28 with 95% CI 1.00–1.64) [39]. Querying the Food and Drug Administration

(FDA) Adverse Event Reporting System, McKenna et al. also noted that there was an increased odds of melanoma for IBD patients on anti-TNF monotherapy and for those who received combination therapy with thiopurines [54].

However, there is an equally if not stronger and more compelling collection of data to show that there is no increased risk for melanomas in patients exposed to anti-TNF therapy. A population-based cohort study from Denmark in 2012 that included more than 56,000 IBD patients who were followed for a median of 3.7 years found no increased risk for any cancers including melanomas [44]. Another population-based study of IBD patients in Olmsted County, Minnesota, diagnosed between 1940 and 2004 by the Mayo Clinic researchers reported no cases of melanoma were found in patients treated with anti-TNF inhibitor [55]. The TREAT registry's prospectively collected data also revealed that there is no increased incidence of melanoma in Crohn's patients treated with infliximab when compared to other treatment groups and the SEER database [43].

NMSC

There are also conflicting results on whether use of anti-TNF inhibitors increases the risk of NMSC. A 2–3-fold increase in risk was observed in Crohn's patients who had recent ($\leq$90 days) or persistent (>365 days) use of TNF monotherapy or combination therapy [37]. Although a subsequent study by Long and colleagues using a different insurance claims database in 2012 came to the opposite conclusion, there was no increased risk after all [39]. An increased risk for NMSC was also found in a query of the FDA Adverse Event Reporting System for anti-TNF inhibitors [54]. Interestingly, a meta-analysis that pooled data from randomized control trials for adalimumab in patients with Crohn's disease found no increase in NMSC risk on TNF monotherapy SIR 1.2 with 95% CI 0.39–2.80 [56].

After reviewing the available data, the risk of either melanomas or NMSC in IBD patients is not likely to be increased above the general population after exposure to anti-TNF alpha therapy as it was previously believed to be [57]. It should be noted that some older studies did not distinguish between patients on anti-TNF therapy who had prior exposure to antimetabolite therapy versus those who were naïve to it. The use of prior antimetabolite therapy is a known risk factor for the development of NMSC.

Thiopurines

Melanomas

There are very few studies to address the question of whether thiopurines increase the risk for melanoma development. Prospectively collected data from Cancers Et Surrisue Associé aux Maladies inflammatories intestinales En France (CESAME) cohort showed that there was no associated increased risk for melanomas in patient who were receiving thiopurines (SIR 1.09 with 95% CI 0.13–3.94), and interestingly, it also showed that there was no increase in risk for patients who had previously been exposed to thiopurines [58]. Long and colleagues' retrospective study examining insurance claims data also noted no increased risk for melanoma in IBD patients on thiopurines (OR 1.10 with 95% CI 0.72–1.67) [39]. On the other hand, Yadav and colleagues observed an association between melanomas and the use of IMM, which in this study included azathioprine and 6-mercaptopurine among other medications [55]. When they examined the Olmsted County cohort's risk, they determined that there was an IRR of 5.3 (with 95% CI 1.1–24.8) although it is not clear how much of that increased risk could be attributed to thiopurines only compared to the other IMM as the researchers did not include a breakdown of the frequency of exposure for each individual IMM [55]. One of the strengths of this retrospective study was that it had a long median follow-up of 18 years.

NMSC

There have been multiple studies published over the past decade that clearly link NMSC and thiopurine exposure together [37–39, 56, 59–61]. IBD patients who take thiopurines have at least a twofold greater risk of developing NMSC when compared to general population [37, 39, 62]. Younger age of exposure confers a greater risk when compared to older age of exposure [62]. We have also learned that longer cumulative duration of thiopurine exposure increases one's risk for the development of NMSC [37, 62, 63]. Although the data is conflicting, that risk may decrease but is not perceived to return to baseline upon discontinuation of thiopurine therapy [55, 61–63].

It is not clear that exposure to thiopurines leads to an increased risk for melanomas, but there is no doubt that thiopurine use is associated with increased risk for NMSC.

Methods to Help Decrease the Risk of Skin Cancers Among IBD Patients

(i) Sun-protective measures – It is recommended that IBD patients, similar to the general population, should engage in avoidance of artificial or natural ultraviolet (UV) light or use a broad-spectrum sunscreen that is protective against UVA and UVB light with a sun protection factor (SPF) of 30 or greater [35, 64]. Reapplication of sunscreen should be done at least every 2 hours if continuous exposure to UV rays is expected [64]. Additionally, patients should routinely wear sun-protective clothing that cover the exposed skin as well as hats and sunglasses [64].

(ii) Skin exam – In the recently published preventative care guidelines for IBD patients by the American College of Gastroenterology (ACG), a skin exam performed by a dermatologist is recommended on initiation of immunosuppressive therapy [35]. Timing of subsequent skin exams for surveillance should then be individualized based on each patient's risk factors [35]. The guideline also suggests that IBD patients maintained on thiopurine therapy who are 50 years or older should receive skin exam to screen for NMSC based on data from the CESAME group that indicated there was an increased risk after that age. CESAME group found that before the age of 50, the incidence of NMSC in patients who were taking thiopurines was 0.66/1000 patient-years, while those who were previously on thiopurines had an incidence of 0.38/1000 patient-years [65]. They also found that from age 50 to 65, the incidences of NMSC in patients who were taking thiopurines and those had been on it previously were 2.59/1000 patient-years and 1.96/1000 patient-years, respectively, and beyond the age of 65, the incidence was greater at 4.04/1000 patient-years and 5.70/1000 patient-years, respectively [65]. However, it is important for IBD patients to continue to receive regular skin exams even after immunosuppressive therapy is later discontinued since it is not clear that their risk for skin cancer decreases or return to a baseline population risk [35]. The recommendation for patients to receive regular skin exams, performed by a physician or themselves, is not based upon data from any randomized control trials, but given the known increased risk for skin cancer on immunosuppressive therapy, it makes sense to engage IBD patients in measures to allow for early detection, rapid referral to dermatology for diagnosis, and treatment of a skin cancer [35].

A recent cost-effective analysis for skin exams showed that they can be effective but costly tool for skin cancer surveillance [66]. The authors found that it is more cost-effective for patients to undergo a skin exam every other year compared to annual surveillance. The same group also showed that there is currently a low rate of adherence to skin cancer screening in IBD patients from their center. Even though 21.3% of their IBD patients had a healthcare encounter with a dermatologist, only 2.6% had at least one total body exam during the study period [67].

(iii) Education on skin cancer risk – Patients should be informed about their individual risk factors for developing a skin cancer and counseled on appropriate preventative measures [35]. One survey-based study performed at a tertiary care center showed that while IBD patients are generally aware of a link between IBD and skin cancer, they lacked knowledge pertaining to prevention, protection, and sun exposure practices [68]. This study highlights a crucial area of IBD patient care that needs further improvement. Development of better methods to convey important educational information regarding skin cancer risk and preventive measures is critical to help bridge this large gap in patient knowledge.

References

1. Jacobson CA, Longo DL. Non-Hodgkin's lymphoma. In: Jameson J, Fauci AS, Kasper DL, Hauser SL, Longo DL, Loscalzo J, editors. Harrison's principles of internal medicine, 20e. New York: McGraw-Hill. http://accessmedicine.mhmedical.com/content.aspx?bookid=2129&sectionid=192018038. Accessed 16 July 2018.
2. Jacobson CA, Longo DL. Hodgkin's lymphoma. In: Jameson J, Fauci AS, Kasper DL, Hauser SL, Longo DL, Loscalzo J, editors. Harrison's principles of internal medicine, 20e. New York: McGraw-Hill. http://accessmedicine.mhmedical.com/content.aspx?bookid=2129&sectionid=192018130. Accessed 16 July 2018.
3. The National Cancer Institute: Surveillance, Epidemiology, and End Results Program (2018). https://seer.cancer.gov/. Accessed 23 July 2018.
4. American Cancer Society: Lymphoma (2018). https://www.cancer.org/cancer/lymphoma.html. Accessed 23 July 2018.
5. Bargen JA. Chronic ulcerative colitis associated with malignant disease. Arch Surg. 1928;17:561–76.
6. Greenstein AJ, Gennuso R, Sachar DB, Heimann T, Smith H, Janowitz HD, et al. Extraintestinal cancers in inflammatory bowel disease. Cancer. 1985;56:2914–21. https://doi.org/10.1002/1097-0142(19851215)56:12<2914::AID-CNCR2820561232>3.0.CO;2-J.
7. Masel S, Hanauer S. Increased association of lymphoma and inflammatory bowel disease. Gastroenterology. 2000;118:A119.
8. Farrell RJ, Ang Y, Kileen P, O'Briain DS, Kelleher D, Keeling PWN, et al. Increased incidence of non-Hodgkin's lymphomas in inflammatory bowel disease patients on immunosuppressive therapy but overall risk is low. Gut. 2000;47:514–9.
9. Ekbom A, Helmick C, Zack M, Adami HO. Extracolonic malignancies in inflammatory bowel disease. Cancer. 1991;67:2015–9.
10. Persson PG, Karlen P, Bernell O, Leijonmarck CE, Brostom O, Ahlbom A, et al. Crohn's disease and cancer: a population-based cohort study. Gastroenterology. 1994;107:1675–9.
11. Karlen P, Lofberg R, Brostrom O, Leijonmarck CE, Helllers G, Persson PG. Increased risk of cancer in ulcerative colitis: a population-based cohort study. Am J Gastroenterol. 1999;94:1047–52.
12. Winther KV, Jess T, Langholz E, Munkholm P, Binder V. Long-term risk of cancer in ulcerative colitis: a population-based cohort study from Copenhagen County. Clin Gastroenterol Hepatol. 2004;2(2):1088–95.
13. Jess T, Winther KV, Munkholm P, Langholz E, Binder V. Intestinal and extra-intestinal cancer in Crohn's disease: follow-up of a population-based cohort in Copenhagen County. Denmark Aliment Pharmacrol Ther. 2004;19:287–93.
14. Beaugerie L, Brousse N, Bouvier AM, Colombel JF, Lemann M, Cosnes J, et al. Lymphoproliferative disorders in patients receiving thiopurines for inflammatory bowel disease: a prospective observational cohort study. Lancet. 2009;374:1617–25.
15. Sokol H, Beaugerie L. Inflammatory bowel disease and lymphoproliferative disorders: the dust is starting to settle. Gut. 2009;58:1427–36.
16. Vos ACW, Bakkal N, Minnee RC, Casparie MK, de Jong DJ, Dijkstra G, et al. Risk of malignant lymphoma in patients with inflammatory bowel diseases: a Dutch nationwide study. Inflamm Bowel Dis. 2011;17:1837–45.
17. Loftus EV Jr, Tremaine WJ, Habermann TM, Harmsen WS, Zinsmeister AR, Sandborn WJ. Risk of lymphoma in inflammatory bowel disease. Am J Gastroenterol. 2000;95(9):2308–12.
18. Lewis JD, Bilker WB, Brensinger C, Deren JJ, Vaughn DJ, Strom BL. Inflammatory bowel disease is not associated with an increased risk of lymphoma. Gastroenterology. 2001;121:1080–7.

19. Askling J, Brandt L, Lapidus A, Karlen P, Bjorkholm M, Lofberg R, et al. Risk of haematopoietic cancer in patients with inflammatory bowel disease. Gut. 2005;54:617–22.
20. Bernstein CN, Blanchard JF, Kliewer E, Wajda A. Cancer risk in patients with inflammatory bowel disease: a population-based study. Cancer. 2001;91:854–62.
21. Palli D, Trallori G, Bagnoli S, Saieva C, Tarantino O, Ceroti M, et al. Hodgkin's disease risk is increased in patients with ulcerative colitis. Gastroenterology. 2000;119:647–53.
22. Loftus EV Jr. Lymphoma risk in inflammatory bowel disease: influences of referral bias and therapy. Gastroenterology. 2001;121:1240–1.
23. Jones JL, Loftus EV Jr. Lymphoma risk in inflammatory bowel disease: is it the disease or the treatment? Inflamm Bowel Dis. 2007;13:1299–307.
24. Bewtra M. Lymphoma in inflammatory bowel disease and treatment decisions. Am J Gastroenterol. 2012;107:964–70.
25. Subramaniam K, D'Rozario J, Pavli P. Lymphoma and other lymphoproliferative disorders in inflammatory bowel disease: a review. J Gastroenterol Hepatol. 2013;28(1):24–30.
26. American Cancer Society. Cancer facts and figures (2018). https://www.cancer.org/content/dam/cancer-org/research/cancer-facts-and-statistics/annual-cancer-facts-and-figures/2018/cancer-facts-and-figures-2018.pdf. Accessed 23 July 2018.
27. American Cancer Society. Melanoma skin cancer (2018). https://www.cancer.org/cancer/melanoma-skin-cancer.html. Accessed 23 July 2018.
28. Curti BD, Leachman S, Urba WJ. Cancer of the skin. In: Jameson J, Fauci AS, Kasper DL, Hauser SL, Longo DL, Loscalzo J, editors. Harrison's principles of internal medicine, 20e. New York: McGraw-Hill. http://accessmedicine.mhmedical.com/content.aspx?bookid=2129&sectionid=192015390. Accessed 16 July 2018.
29. Rogers HW, Weinstock MA, Feldman SR, Coldiron BM. Incidence estimate of nonmelanoma skin cancer (keratinocyte carcinomas) in the US population, 2012. JAMA Dermatol. 2015;151(10):1081–6.
30. World Health Organization. Skin cancers. http://www.who.int/uv/faq/skincancer/en/index2.html. Accessed 23 July 2018.
31. Skin Cancer Foundation. Skin cancer facts & statistics. https://www.skincancer.org/skin-cancer-information/skin-cancer-facts. Accessed 23 July 2018.
32. Marcil I, Stern RS. Risk of developing a subsequent nonmelanoma skin cancer in patients with a history of nonmelanoma skin cancer: a critical review of the literature and meta-analysis. Arch Dermatol. 2000;136(12):1524–30.
33. Singh S, Nagpal SJS, Murad MH, Yadav S, Kane SV, Pardi DS, et al. Inflammatory bowel disease is associated with an increased risk of melanoma: a systematic review and meta-analysis. Clin Gastroenterol Hepatol. 2014;12:210–8.
34. Nissen LHC, Pierik M, Derikx LAAP, de Jong E, Kievit W, van den Heuvel TR, et al. Risk factors and clinical outcomes in patients with IBD with melanoma. Inflamm Bowel Dis. 2017;23:2018–26.
35. Farraye FA, Melmed GY, Lichtenstein GR, Kane SV. ACG clinical guideline: preventative care in inflammatory bowel disease. Am J Gastroenterol. 2017;112:241–58.
36. Mellemkjaer L, Olsen JH, Frisch M, Johansen C, Gridley G, McLaughlin JK. Cancer in patients with ulcerative colitis. Ing J Cancer. 1995;60:330–3.
37. Long MD, Herfarth HH, Pipkin C, Porter CQ, Sandler RS, Kappelman M. Increased risk for non-melanoma skin cancer in patients with inflammatory bowel disease. Clin Gastroenterol Hepatol. 2010;8(3):268–74.
38. Singh H, Nugent Z, Demers AA, Bernstein CN. Increased risk of nonmelanoma skin cancers among individuals with inflammatory bowel disease. Gastroenterology. 2011;141:1612–20.
39. Long MD, Martin CF, Pipkin CA, Herfarth HH, Sandler RS, Kappelman MD. Risk of melanoma and nonmelanoma skin cancer among patients with inflammatory bowel disease. Gastroenterology. 2012;143(3):390–9.
40. Lemaitre M, Kirchgesner J, Rudnichi A, Carrat F, Zureik M, Carbonnel F, et al. Association between use of thiopurines or tumor necrosis factor antagonists alone or in combination and risk of lymphoma in patients with inflammatory bowel disease. JAMA. 2017;318(17):1679–86.

41. Khan N, Abbas AM, Lichtenstein GR, Loftus EV Jr, Bazzano LA. Risk of lymphoma in patients with ulcerative colitis treated with thiopurines: a nationwide retrospective cohort study. Gastroenterology. 2013;145(5):1007–15.
42. Kotlyar DS, Lewis JD, Beaugerie L, Tierney A, Brensinger CM, Gisbert JP, et al. Risk of lymphoma in patients with inflammatory bowel disease treated with azathioprine and 6-mercaptopurine: a meta-analysis. Clin Gastroenterol Hepatol. 2015;13(5):847–58.
43. Lichtenstein GR, Feagan BG, Cohen RD, Salzberg BA, Diamond RH, Langholff W, et al. Drug therapies and the risk of malignancy in Crohn's disease: results from the TREAT™ registry. Am J Gastroenterol. 2014;109:212–23.
44. Nyboe Andersen N, Pasternak B, Basit S, Andersson M, Svanstrom H, Capsersen S, et al. Association between tumor necrosis factor-α antagonists and risk of cancer in patients with inflammatory bowel disease. JAMA. 2014;311(23):2406–13.
45. Herrinton LJ, Liu L, Weng X, Lewis JD, Hutfless S, Allison JE. Role of thiopurine and anti-TNF therapy in lymphoma in inflammatory bowel disease. Am J Gastroenterol. 2011;106(12):2146–53.
46. Siegel CA, Marden SM, Persing SM, Larson RJ, Sands BE. Risk of lymphoma associated with combination anti-tumor necrosis factor and immunomodulator therapy for the treatment of Crohn's disease: a meta-analysis. Clin Gastroenterol Hepatol. 2009;7:874–81.
47. Farrell RJ, Ang Y, Kileen P, O'Briain DS, Kelleher D, Keeling PW, et al. Increased incidence of non-Hodgkin's lymphoma in inflammatory bowel disease patients on immunosuppressive therapy but overall risk is low. Gut. 2000;47:514–9.
48. Curtis JR, Lee EB, Kaplan IV, Kwok K, Geier J, Benda B, et al. Tofacitinib, an oral Janus kinase inhibitor: analysis of malignancies across the rheumatoid arthritis clinical development programme. Ann Rheum Dis. 2016;75(5):831–41.
49. Sandborn WJ, Su C, Sands BE, D'Haens GR, Vermeire S, Schreiber S, et al. Tofacitinib as induction and maintenance therapy for ulcerative colitis. N Engl J Med. 2017;376(18):1723–36.
50. Lichtenstein GR, Loftus EV, Bloom S, Lawendy N, Friedman GS, Zhang H, et al. Tofacitinib, an Oral Janus kinase inhibitor, in the treatment of ulcerative colitis: open-label, Long-term extension study. Poster presentation Digestive Diseases Week. October 2017.
51. Feagan BG, Sandborn WJ, Gasink C, Jacobstein D, Lang Y, Friedman JR, et al. Ustekinumab as induction and maintenance therapy for Crohn's disease. N Engl J Med. 2016;375(20):1946–60.
52. Amiot A, Serrero M, Peyrin-Biroulet L, Filippi J, Pariente B, Roblin X, et al. One-year effectiveness and safety of vedolizumab therapy for inflammatory bowel disease: a prospective multicentre cohort study. Aliment Pharmacol Ther. 2017;46(3):310–21.
53. Bye WA, Jairath V, Travis SPL. Systematic review: the safety of vedolizumab for the treatment of inflammatory bowel disease. Aliment Pharmacol Ther. 2017;46(1):3–15.
54. McKenna MR, Stobaugh DJ, Deepak P. Melanoma and non-melanoma skin cancer in inflammatory bowel disease patients following tumor necrosis factor-α inhibitor monotherapy and in combination with thiopurines: analysis of the food and drug administration adverse event reporting system. J Gastrointestin Liv Dis. 2014;23(3):267–71.
55. Yadav S, Singh S, Harmsen WS, Varayil JE, Tremaine WJ, Loftus EV Jr. Effects of medications on risk of cancer in patients with inflammatory bowel diseases: a population-based cohort study from Olmsted County. Minnesota Mayo Clin Proc. 2015;90(6):738–46.
56. Osterman MT, Sandborn WJ, Colombel JF, Robinson AM, Lau W, Huang B, et al. Increased risk of malignancy with adalimumab combination therapy, compared with monotherapy, for Crohn's disease. Gastroenterology. 2014;146(4):941–9.
57. Cohn HM, Dave M, Loftus EV Jr. Understanding the cautions and contraindications of immunomodulator and biologic therapies for use in inflammatory bowel disease. Inflamm Bowel Dis. 2017;23(8):1301–15.
58. Peyrin-Biroulet L, Chevaux JB, Bouvier AM, Carrat F, Beaugerie L. Risk of melanoma in patients who receive thiopurines for inflammatory bowel disease is not increased. Am J Gastroenterol. 2012;107:1443–4.
59. Ariyaratnam J, Subramanian V. Association between thiopurine use and nonmelanoma skin cancers in patients with inflammatory bowel disease: a meta-analysis. Am J Gastroenterol. 2014;109:163–9.

60. Scott FI, Mamtani R, Brensinger CM, Haynes K, Chiesa-Fuxench Z, Zhang J, et al. Risk of nonmelanoma skin cancer associated with the use of immunosuppressant and biologic agents in patients with a history of autoimmune disease and nonmelanoma skin cancer. JAMA Dermatol. 2016;152(2):164–72.
61. Hagen JW, Pugliano-Mauro MA. Nonmelanoma skin cancer risk in patients with inflammatory bowel disease undergoing thiopurine therapy: a systematic review of the literature. Dermatol Surg. 2018;44(4):469–80.
62. Abbas AM, Almuktar RM, Loftus EV Jr, Lichenstein GR, Khan N. Risk of melanoma and non-melanoma skin cancer in ulcerative colitis patients treated with thiopurines: a nationwide retrospective cohort. Am J Gastroenterol. 2014;109(11):1781–93.
63. Kopylov U, Vutcovici M, Kezouh A, Seidman E, Bitton A, Afif W. Risk of lymphoma, colorectal and skin cancer in patients with IBD treated with immunomodulators and biologics: a Quebec claims database study. Inflamm Bowel Dis. 2015;21:1847–53.
64. Long MD, Kappelman MD, Pipkin CA. Non-melanoma skin cancer in inflammatory bowel disease: a review. Inflamm Bowel Dis. 2011;17(6):1423–7.
65. Peyrin-Biroulet L, Khosrotehrani K, Carrat F, Bouvier AM, Chevaux JB, Simon T, et al. Increased risk for nonmelanoma skin cancers in patients who receive thiopurines for inflammatory bowel disease. Gastroenterology. 2011;141(5):1621–8.
66. Anderson AJ, Ferris LK, Binion DG, Smith KJ. Cost-effectiveness of melanoma screening in inflammatory bowel disease. Dig Dis Sci. 2018;63(10):2564–72.
67. Anderson AJ, Ferris LK, Click B, Ramos-Rivera C, Koutroubakis IE, Hashash JG, et al. Low rates of dermatologic care and skin cancer screening among inflammatory bowel disease patients. Dig Dis Sci. 2018;63(10):2729–39.
68. Kimmel JN, Taft TH, Keefer L. Inflammatory bowel disease and skin cancer: an assessment of patient risk factors, knowledge and skin practices. J Skin Cancer. 2016;2016:4632037.

Chapter 9
Preventing Colorectal Cancer in Patients with Inflammatory Bowel Diseases: Chemopreventive and Surgical Approaches

Siddharth Singh

Background

Patients with inflammatory bowel diseases (IBDs) are at increased risk of colorectal cancer (CRC). Though the risks were potentially overestimated in early studies, more recent population-based study cohorts continue to demonstrate a 1.1–5.3% cumulative risk of CRC at 20 years, with a 2.4 times higher risk than the general population [1].

The pathophysiology of IBD-associated CRC is different than the pathophysiology of more typical, sporadic CRC [2]. While sporadic CRC is caused by a series of random mutations in either the APC gene pathway or the MSH gene pathway, IBD-associated CRC may be related to the chronic inflammatory state caused by IBD and exhibits a different set of genetic mutations. There are four primary pathogenic factors that contribute to IBD-associated CRC. First, chronic uncontrolled inflammation itself may result in neoplastic transformation by increasing cell turnover in the colonic epithelium increasing the probability of replicative errors. Mucosal biopsies of areas of active inflammation demonstrate high rates of mitosis and apoptosis. Chronic inflammation results in high levels of pro-inflammatory cytokines within the colonic mucosa (e.g., tumor necrosis factor-alpha [TNF-a], interleukin-6 [IL-6], interleukin-10 [IL-10], interferon-gamma [IFN-g]), leading to the activation of several transcription factors involved in cancer development. At a molecular level, IL-6 promotes tumor growth and inhibits apoptosis by activating the JAK/

S. Singh (✉)
Division of Gastroenterology, University of California San Diego, La Jolla, CA, USA

Division of Biomedical Informatics, Department of Medicine, University of California San Diego, La Jolla, CA, USA
e-mail: sis040@ucsd.edu

© Springer Nature Switzerland AG 2019
J. D. Feuerstein, A. S. Cheifetz (eds.), *Cancer Screening in Inflammatory Bowel Disease*, https://doi.org/10.1007/978-3-030-15301-4_9

STAT signaling pathway. Cyclooxygenase-2 (COX-2) overexpression occurs early in, mainly due to pro-inflammatory cytokines IL-1 and TNF-a, leading to cell proliferation, angiogenesis, and apoptosis. Second, unique gene products are highly expressed in both inflamed mucosa and CRC. Oxidative stress, increased in IBD due to chronic inflammation and increased phagocytosis by leukocytes, has also been linked to malignancy. More recent studies suggest that commensal microbiota may also have an impact on carcinogenesis and tumor progression, through a complex interaction between diet, bile acids, and the immune system [3]. Dysbiosis has been implicated in cancer-associated inflammation, by activating survival genes within neoplastic cells and pro-inflammatory genes in the tumor microenvironment.

Risk Factors for IBD-Associated Colorectal Cancer

Several risk factors have been associated with increased risk of CRC. Non-modifiable risk factors include coexistent primary sclerosing cholangitis (PSC), long disease duration, extensive colitis, young age at diagnosis, and family history of colorectal cancer [2, 4]. Important modifiable risk factors for IBD-associated CRC are smoking and uncontrolled inflammation. Counseling for smoking cessation is a foregone conclusion in all patients with IBD. High cumulative burden of inflammation is also an independent and strong risk factor for IBD-associated CRC. In a single-center cohort study of 987 patients followed over 13 years, Choi and colleagues observed that cumulative inflammatory burden (defined as sum of average score between each pair of surveillance episodes multiplied by the surveillance interval in years) was significantly associated with risk of colorectal neoplasia development (hazard ratio, 2.1 per 10-unit increase in cumulative inflammatory burden [equivalent of 10, 5, or 3.3 years of continuous mild, moderate, or severe active microscopic inflammation]; 95% CI, 1.4–3.0) [5]. While inflammation severity based on the most recent colonoscopy alone was not significant (HR, 0.9 per-1-unit increase in severity), a mean severity score calculated from all colonoscopies performed in preceding 5 years was significantly associated with the risk of colorectal neoplasia (HR, 2.2 per-1-unit increase; 95% CI, 1.6–3.1).

Based on this risk of colorectal neoplasia, and known risk factors, routine surveillance for colorectal cancer has been recommended in patients with IBD, despite the lack of adequately controlled prospective studies to formally evaluate the benefits, risks, and costs of this approach [6, 7]. Suboptimal adherence, access, and expense limit population-wide adoption of colonoscopy for CRC prevention. Additionally, despite routine screening, a fraction of individuals still develop interval CRC before their recommended surveillance interval, either due to missed or incompletely resected lesions or rapidly growing tumors.

Chemoprevention Against IBD-Associated Colorectal Cancer

Given the limitations of screening tests and poor prognosis associated with advanced stage CRC, there is great interest in exploring chemoprevention strategies to reduce the burden of this preventable malignancy [8, 9]. No chemopreventive agent has been tested in an interventional study in patients with IBD, and all information has been obtained from cohort studies with inherent limitations of an observational design.

Chemopreventive agents in patients with IBD may be divided into two classes: first, those directly used in treatment of IBD (5-aminosalicylates, thiopurines, tumor necrosis factor-α antagonists) and second, those not directly related to IBD, which may have an independent chemopreventive effect (aspirin, folic acid, ursodeoxycholic acid).

IBD Therapies as Chemopreventive Agents

5-Aminosalicylic Acid

5-Aminosalicylic acid (5-ASA) is the most commonly used medication for the treatment of ulcerative colitis. Although their mechanism of chemoprevention is speculative, several theories have been proposed including a role in reducing oxidative stress, inhibiting cell proliferation, and promoting apoptosis [10]. 5-ASA also seems to be an inhibitor of a variety of pro-inflammatory cytokines that can lead to malignancy in mouse models including TNF-α, NF-κB, transforming growth factor-beta (TGF-β), and Wnt/β-catenin.

In a meta-analysis of nine observational studies, Velayos and colleagues observed that 5-ASA exposure was associated with a 49% lower risk of colorectal neoplasia (OR, 0.51; 95% CI, 0.37–0.69), with lower risk observed with longer duration of therapy, with a dose–response relationship [11]. However, contradictory results have been observed in non-referral center, population-based studies. Jess et al. conducted a nested case–control study in a cohort of patients from Copenhagen, Denmark, and Olmsted County, Minnesota [12]. Of 1160 Danish and 692 Minnesotan IBD patients, a total of 26 patients were identified who had developed CRC. Control patients were matched for several confounding factors. Daily (>1.2 g/day) and cumulative dose (per 1000 g) of mesalamine were not associated with a significant reduction in the rate of CRC (OR, 1.6; 95% CI, 0.3–7.1 and OR, 1.3; 95% CI, 0.9–1.9, respectively). In a meta-analysis of four non-referral studies including 608 patients with CRC and 2177 controls, Nguyen and colleagues concluded that 5-ASA use was not associated with the reduced risk of CRC in patients with IBD (OR, 0.95; 95% CI, 0.66–1.38) [13]. These contradictory results could be due to inherent biases in referral centers.

Based on this, the true independent effect of 5-ASA on CRC risk in patients with IBD is unclear. The European Crohn's and Colitis Organization guidelines for UC management include a statement suggesting 5-ASA compounds should be considered for all UC patients for their possible chemopreventive effect, but this is not reflected by other societies [6, 14]. In the author's opinion, 5-ASA should be used for the treatment of UC in patients with mild to moderate disease; however, it should not be used for the primary purpose of chemoprevention, in patients who have otherwise failed 5-ASA, or in patients with colonic Crohn's disease.

Thiopurines

Thiopurines are effective medications for maintenance of remission in patients with IBD and are frequently used either as monotherapy or in combination with biologic agents to prevent disease-related complications. By acting as purine antagonists and interference with the synthesis of DNA, RNA, and a number of pro-inflammatory proteins, they may have putative cancer prevention effect. Downregulation of activated T cells through DNA intercalation leads to reductions in the transcription of TNF-related apoptosis-inducing ligand, TNF receptor superfamily member 7, and α-4 integrin [9]. Thiopurines also inhibit Rac1, leading to an acceleration of T-cell apoptosis.

Thiopurines have been consistently associated with an increased risk of hematological malignancies and non-melanoma skin cancers [2]. However, by controlling inflammation effectively, they may be associated with decreasing the risk of colorectal cancer. In two population-based studies, no significant association has been observed between thiopurine use and risk of CRC. In a propensity-matched population-based cohort study of 45,986 patients with IBD (median follow-up, 7.9 years; median duration of azathioprine use in those exposed, 1.9 years), Pasternak et al. observed that there was no difference in the risk of CRC between current (RR, 1.36; 95% CI, 0.75–2.49) and former thiopurine users (RR, 0.71; 95% CI, 0.34–1.46) vs. nonusers [15]. However, in a recent meta-analysis of 24 studies with 76,999 patients, Lu and colleagues observed a lower risk of colorectal neoplasia (OR, 0.63; 95% CI, 0.46–0.86), advanced colorectal neoplasia (CRC and/or high-grade dysplasia) (OR, 0.62; 95% CI, 0.44–0.89), and CRC (OR, 0.65; 95% CI, 0.45–0.96) with the use of thiopurines in patients with IBD [16].

There are no specific guidelines addressing the role of thiopurines for cancer prevention in IBD. In the author's opinion, as for 5-ASA, thiopurine use should be determined based on active IBD, and these medications should not be used solely for prevention of CRC.

Tumor Necrosis Factor-α Antagonists

TNFα antagonists are one of the most effective medications for treatment of moderate to severe IBD. Like thiopurines, TNFα antagonists have also been variably associated with increased risk of lymphoma, but not other solid organ cancers. The

TNFα pathway results in the production of NF-κB and activation of COX-2 which may lead to cancer, and hence, theoretically TNFα antagonists may decrease the risk of cancer [9].

There are a small number of studies examining the use of TNFα antagonists and risk of CRC in patients with IBD. In an observational study examining the long-term safety of infliximab in Belgium, none of 734 IBD patients on infliximab developed CRC, as compared to 8/666 patients without exposure to infliximab [17]. In another study utilizing a nationwide database in the Netherlands, 173 IBD patients diagnosed with CRC were identified and matched with 393 control patients [18]. Use of infliximab was highly protective against the development of CRC (OR, 0.09; 95% CI, 0.01–0.68). However, limited population-based studies have shown conflicting results. In a Danish nationwide registry following over 50,000 patients for almost 500,000 person-years (median 9.3 years) and compared the rates of a several cancers between TNFα antagonists-exposed (8.1% of the cohort) vs. TNFα antagonists-naïve patients, TNFα antagonist use was not associated with a reduced risk of CRC (OR, 1.0; 95% CI, 0.48–2.08) [19].

Based on above, and inherent side effects and costs of TNFα antagonists, they are not recommended solely for chemoprevention even in high-risk patients. There is very limited data on newer non-TNF biologics in modifying risk of CRC. We anticipate that by effectively controlling mucosal inflammation, their use will also be associated with lower risk of CRC.

Chemopreventive Effects of Other Therapies

Ursodeoxycholic Acid

Secondary bile acids in stool, including deoxycholic acid and lithocholic acid, may play an important role in the pathogenesis of CRC, through disruption of the balance between colorectal crypt cell proliferation, differentiation, and apoptosis. Ursodeoxycholic acid (UDCA), the 7-β-epimer of chenodeoxycholic acid that is used in patients with chronic cholestatic diseases such as PSC, has been shown to have a chemopreventive effect based on in vitro and animal models [20].

Clinical studies evaluating the role of UDCA in preventing IBD-associated colorectal neoplasia (CRC and/or high-grade dysplasia [HGD] and/or low-grade dysplasia [LGD]) have shown conflicting results. In a meta-analysis of eight studies (five observational, three randomized controlled trials) reporting 177 cases of colorectal neoplasia in 763 patients with PSC-IBD, we observed a significant protective association between UDCA use and advanced colorectal neoplasia (CRC and/or high-grade dysplasia) (OR, 0.35; 95% CI, 0.17–0.73), but not all colorectal neoplasia (OR, 0.81; 95% CI, 0.41–1.61) [20]. In a subgroup analysis, low-dose UDCA use (8–15 mg/kg/day) was associated with significant risk reduction of colorectal neoplasia (OR, 0.19; 95% CI, 0.08–0.49), whereas doses between 15 and 30 mg/kg/day did not modify the risk of colorectal neoplasia in three studies.

Based on these findings, there are discrepant recommendations from clinical societies. The American Association for the Study of Liver Diseases recommends against the use of UDCA among patients with PSC-IBD for CRC prevention, whereas the European Association for the Study of the Liver recommends that UDCA may be considered in high-risk groups such as those with a strong family history of CRC, previous colorectal dysplasia, or long-standing extensive colitis. In the authors' opinion, low-dose UDCA if used for treating PSC may have a favorable effect on CRC prevention; however, in the absence of a prospective chemoprevention trial or modeling studies of cost–benefit ratio, it should not be used primarily for the purposes of chemoprevention in patients with PSC-IBD.

Other Chemopreventive Agents (Aspirin, NSAIDs, Folic Acid, Statins)

Aspirin, other NSAIDs, and statins have been investigated for their anti-inflammatory effects in other diseases as well as sporadic CRC. While none of these medications have any effect as a primary treatment for IBD, there is a plausible biologic basis for a possible effect in reducing the risk of IBD-associated CRC including reducing prostaglandin production by inhibition of COX-2 activity and inhibition of HMG-CoA activity. In a network meta-analysis of 14 chemoprevention trials comparing 10 different treatment strategies in patients with prior sporadic colorectal neoplasia, we observed that non-aspirin NSAIDs may be effective for the prevention of advanced metachronous neoplasia over a 3- to 5-year period, but the risk-to-benefit profile potentially favors its use only in individuals with a history of high-risk neoplasia [21]. After non-aspirin NSAIDs, low-dose aspirin alone had the second highest probability of being most effective for preventing advanced metachronous neoplasia, and with its favorable risk-to-benefit profile, it may be considered as secondary colorectal cancer chemoprevention agent in a select group of patients. Other therapies including vitamin D, calcium, folic acid alone, or in combination were not effective for decreasing the risk of advanced metachronous neoplasia.

There has been limited evaluation of these medications for chemoprevention in patients with IBD. In a meta-analysis of eight observational studies of non-aspirin NSAIDs and three studies of aspirin, there was no significant association between exposure to either medication and risk of IBD-associated CRC (non-aspirin NSAIDs, OR, 0.80; 95% CI, 0.39–1.21; aspirin, OR, 0.66; 95% CI, 0.06–1.39) [22]. In contrast, statin exposure may be associated with a lower risk of IBD-associated CRC. In a larger retrospective cohort study of 1376 IBD patients, exposure to statins was associated with lower risk of developing CRC over 9 years of follow-up (OR, 0.42; 95% CI, 0.28–0.62) [23]. Similarly, folic acid supplementation was also associated with 42% lower risk of CRC in a meta-analysis of ten retrospective studies in patients with IBD [24].

Based on these findings from observational studies at high risk of measured and unmeasured biases, the author does not recommend routine use of these medications primarily for chemoprevention in patients with IBD. If used for other clear indications, they may have a protective effect.

Surgery for Prevention of Colorectal Cancer in Patients with IBD

With advances in endoscopic dysplasia detection techniques, there has been an increase in the rate of detection of low-grade dysplasia in patients with IBD. Several of these lesions, particularly those with polypoid dysplasia or visible and resectable non-polypoid dysplasia, should be treated endoscopically, and after resection enhanced, surveillance is recommended. However, some dysplastic lesions at high risk of progression to advanced neoplasia may require surgical resection for prevention of progression of dysplasia.

In a comprehensive study of 172 patients with UC with low-grade dysplasia followed for median 4 years, Choi and colleagues made important observations [25]. Overall, 33 patients developed high grade or CRC (during study period). Multivariate Cox proportional hazard analysis revealed that macroscopically non-polypoid (HR, 8.6; 95% CI, 3.0–24.8) or invisible (HR, 4.1; 95% CI, 1.3–13.4) dysplasia, dysplastic lesions ≥1 cm in size (HR, 3.8; 95% CI, 1.5–13.4), and a previous history of "indefinite for dysplasia" (HR, 2.8; 95% CI, 1.2–6.5) were significant contributory factors for HGD or CRC development. They estimated that the risk of progression was higher in patients with multiple risk factor. The cumulative incidence of advanced neoplasia at 1 and 5 years after initial LGD was 0% and 1.8% for no risk factor, 9.6% and 17.7% for one risk factor (HR, 4.9%), and 29.0% and 53.4% for two risk factors (HR, 13.6%). For those with three risk factors, cumulative risk of HGD or CRC development was 61.6% and 80.7% at 1 and 2 years, respectively. In a subsequent meta-analysis of 14 surveillance cohorts of patients with UC with low-grade dysplasia, we estimated the annual incidence of CRC was approximately 0.8% (95% CI, 0.4–1.3); rates of progression to CRC were higher when LGD was diagnosed by at least one expert gastrointestinal pathologist (incidence rate, 1.5%; 95% CI, 0.6–2.4) as compared to a community pathologist without expert confirmation (IR, 0.2%; 95% CI, 0.0–0.4) [26]. Likewise, in patients with invisible dysplasia, the annual incidence of progression to advanced neoplasia was 6.1% (95% CI, 0.9–11.4) and with endoscopically visible dysplasia was 1.0% (95% CI, 0–2.1). We identified that multifocal lesions, endoscopically invisible lesions, lesions located in the distal colon, or those detected in patients with coexistent PSC were associated with higher risk of progression to advanced neoplasia.

In these patients, at high risk of progression to advanced neoplasia, with endoscopically unresectable lesions, surgery with total proctocolectomy with ileal-pouch anal anastomosis (or with end-ileostomy) should be considered to prevention progression to CRC. Since there are significant differences in patients' and physicians' willingness to undergo colectomy for dysplasia risk, shared decision-making is recommended.

In summary, IBD is associated with an increased risk of CRC, with some potentially modifiable risk factors. Cumulative inflammatory burden is one of the strongest and modifiable risk factors. Controlling active inflammation, using effective IBD-related therapy with 5-ASA, thiopurines, and/or biologic agents, would be expected to decrease CRC risk. Current observational studies of 5-ASA, thiopurines, and biologic agents variably suggest lower risk of CRC in treated patients. However, there are inherent biases due to confounding by indication and severity, as well as unmeasured confounding which limits strong interpretation. In the absence of well-designed prospective randomized studies, the data are not robust enough to recommend using these medications purely for chemoprevention. At the same time, it is very unlikely that such a trial will be performed. Other medications, such as aspirin, non-aspirin NSAIDs, statins, and folic acid, have been well-studied for preventing sporadic CRC, with modest benefit with aspirin and non-aspirin NSAIDs. These medications are unlikely to be pursued for a chemopreventive indication against IBD-associated CRC. In a subset of patients with low-grade dysplasia on surveillance colonoscopies, which is not resectable, surgery for preventing progression to advanced neoplasia may be recommended.

Disclosures Dr. Singh is supported by the National Institute of Diabetes and Digestive and Kidney Diseases of the National Institutes of Health under award number K23DK117058, the American College of Gastroenterology Junior Faculty Development Award, and the Crohn's and Colitis Foundation Career Development Award (#404614).

Conflicts of Interest SS received research grants from Pfizer and AbbVie and consulting fees from AbbVie, Takeda, Pfizer, and AMAG Pharmaceuticals.

References

1. Jess T, Rungoe C, Peyrin-Biroulet L. Risk of colorectal cancer in patients with ulcerative colitis: a meta-analysis of population-based cohort studies. Clin Gastroenterol Hepatol. 2012;10(6):639–45.
2. Beaugerie L, Itzkowitz SH. Cancers complicating inflammatory bowel disease. N Engl J Med. 2015;372(15):1441–52.
3. Chen J, Pitmon E, Wang K. Microbiome, inflammation and colorectal cancer. Semin Immunol. 2017;32:43–53.
4. Dulai PS, Sandborn WJ, Gupta S. Colorectal cancer and dysplasia in inflammatory bowel disease: a review of disease epidemiology, pathophysiology, and management. Cancer Prev Res (Phila). 2016;9(12):887–94.
5. Choi CR, Al Bakir I, Ding NJ, Lee GH, Askari A, Warusavitarne J, et al. Cumulative burden of inflammation predicts colorectal neoplasia risk in ulcerative colitis: a large single-centre study. Gut. 2017. pii:gutjnl-2017-314190. https://doi.org/10.1136/gutjnl-2017-314190.

6. Farraye FA, Odze RD, Eaden J, Itzkowitz SH. AGA technical review on the diagnosis and management of colorectal neoplasia in inflammatory bowel disease. Gastroenterology. 2010;138(2):746–74.

7. Annese V, Beaugerie L, Egan L, Biancone L, Bolling C, Brandts C, et al. European evidence-based consensus: inflammatory bowel disease and malignancies. J Crohns Colitis. 2015;9(11):945–65.

8. Lopez A, Pouillon L, Beaugerie L, Danese S, Peyrin-Biroulet L. Colorectal cancer prevention in patients with ulcerative colitis. Best Pract Res Clin Gastroenterol. 2018;32–33:103–9.

9. Ehrlich AC, Patel S, Meillier A, Rothstein RD, Friedenberg FK. Chemoprevention of colorectal cancer in inflammatory bowel disease. Expert Rev Anticancer Ther. 2017;17(3):247–55.

10. Lopez A, Peyrin-Biroulet L. 5-Aminosalicylic acid and chemoprevention: does it work? Dig Dis. 2013;31(2):248–53.

11. Velayos FS, Terdiman JP, Walsh JM. Effect of 5-aminosalicylate use on colorectal cancer and dysplasia risk: a systematic review and meta-analysis of observational studies. Am J Gastroenterol. 2005;100(6):1345–53.

12. Jess T, Loftus EV Jr, Velayos FS, Winther KV, Tremaine WJ, Zinsmeister AR, et al. Risk factors for colorectal neoplasia in inflammatory bowel disease: a nested case-control study from Copenhagen county, Denmark and Olmsted County, Minnesota. Am J Gastroenterol. 2007;102(4):829–36.

13. Nguyen GC, Gulamhusein A, Bernstein CN. 5-aminosalicylic acid is not protective against colorectal cancer in inflammatory bowel disease: a meta-analysis of non-referral populations. Am J Gastroenterol. 2012;107(9):1298–304.

14. Magro F, Gionchetti P, Eliakim R, Ardizzone S, Armuzzi A, Barreiro-de Acosta M, et al. Third European evidence-based consensus on diagnosis and management of ulcerative colitis. Part 1: definitions, diagnosis, extra-intestinal manifestations, pregnancy, cancer surveillance, surgery, and ileo-anal pouch disorders. J Crohns Colitis. 2017;11(6):649–70.

15. Pasternak B, Svanström H, Schmiegelow K, Jess T, Hviid A. Use of azathioprine and the risk of cancer in inflammatory bowel disease. Am J Epidemiol. 2013;177(11):1296–305.

16. Lu MJ, Qiu XY, Mao XQ, Li XT, Zhang HJ. Systematic review with meta-analysis: thiopurines decrease the risk of colorectal neoplasia in patients with inflammatory bowel disease. Aliment Pharmacol Ther. 2018;47(3):318–31.

17. Fidder H, Schnitzler F, Ferrante M, Noman M, Katsanos K, Segaert S, et al. Long-term safety of infliximab for the treatment of inflammatory bowel disease: a single-centre cohort study. Gut. 2009;58(4):501–8.

18. Baars JE, Looman CW, Steyerberg EW, Beukers R, Tan AC, Weusten BL, et al. The risk of inflammatory bowel disease-related colorectal carcinoma is limited: results from a nationwide nested case-control study. Am J Gastroenterol. 2011;106(2):319–28.

19. Nyboe Andersen N, Pasternak B, Basit S, Andersson M, Svanström H, Caspersen S, et al. Association between tumor necrosis factor-α antagonists and risk of cancer in patients with inflammatory bowel disease. JAMA. 2014;311(23):2406–13.

20. Singh S, Khanna S, Pardi DS, Loftus EV Jr, Talwalkar JA. Effect of ursodeoxycholic acid use on the risk of colorectal neoplasia in patients with primary sclerosing cholangitis and inflammatory bowel disease: a systematic review and meta-analysis. Inflamm Bowel Dis. 2013;19(8):1631–8.

21. Dulai PS, Singh S, Marquez E, Khera R, Prokop LJ, Limburg PJ, et al. Chemoprevention of colorectal cancer in individuals with previous colorectal neoplasia: systematic review and network meta-analysis. BMJ. 2016;355:i6188. https://doi.org/10.1136/bmj.i6188.

22. Burr NE, Hull MA, Subramanian V. Does aspirin or non-aspirin non-steroidal anti-inflammatory drug use prevent colorectal cancer in inflammatory bowel disease? World J Gastroenterol. 2016;22(13):3679–86.

23. Ananthakrishnan AN, Cagan A, Cai T, Gainer VS, Shaw SY, Churchill S, et al. Statin use is associated with reduced risk of colorectal cancer in patients with inflammatory bowel diseases. Clin Gastroenterol Hepatol. 2016;14(7):973–9.

24. Burr NE, Hull MA, Subramanian V. Folic acid supplementation may reduce colorectal cancer risk in patients with inflammatory bowel disease: a systematic review and meta-analysis. J Clin Gastroenterol. 2017;51(3):247–53.
25. Choi CH, Ignjatovic-Wilson A, Askari A, Lee GH, Warusavitarne J, Moorghen M, et al. Low-grade dysplasia in ulcerative colitis: risk factors for developing high-grade dysplasia or colorectal cancer. Am J Gastroenterol. 2015;110(10):1461–71.
26. Fumery M, Dulai PS, Gupta S, Prokop LJ, Ramamoorthy S, Sandborn WJ, Singh S. Incidence, risk factors, and outcomes of colorectal cancer in patients with ulcerative colitis with low-grade dysplasia: a systematic review and meta-analysis. Clin Gastroenterol Hepatol. 2017;15(5):665–74.

Chapter 10
Cancer Risk and Screening in Pediatric Patients

Matthew Kowalik and Stacy A. Kahn

Introduction

The topic of cancer is a frequent discussion point in pediatric inflammatory bowel disease (IBD) despite that it remains uncommon. Cancer discussions in pediatric IBD are centered around therapy and surveillance. Although colorectal carcinoma (CRC) is rare in pediatric IBD patients, increased CRC screening by colonoscopy in the pediatric age group has identified several cases [1]. Inflammatory bowel disease has also been associated with extraintestinal cancers; these include blood malignancies such as leukemia, lymphoma, and hepatosplenic T-cell lymphoma (HSTCL), liver cancers, skin cancers (melanoma and nonmelanoma skin cancer [NMSC]), and potentially cervical cancer. Pediatric cancer remains a rare phenomenon, and the body of literature regarding cancer in pediatric IBD is limited. Large prospective studies remain an area of need to help inform treatment guidelines and discussions around risk.

Despite the lack of data regarding cancer in the pediatric IBD population and its rarity, discussions regarding cancer play important role in management. Prior to starting an immunomodulator or biologic, the risk of cancer secondary to therapy is a frequent discussion point for physicians and a serious concern for families. The subject has become exceedingly relevant as the use of immunomodulators and

M. Kowalik
Division of Gastroenterology, Hepatology and Nutrition, Boston Children's Hospital, Boston, MA, USA
e-mail: Matthew.Kowalik@childrens.harvard.edu

S. A. Kahn (✉)
Inflammatory Bowel Disease Center, Boston Children's Hospital, Boston, MA, USA

Harvard Medical School, Boston, MA, USA
e-mail: Stacy.Kahn@childrens.harvard.edu

© Springer Nature Switzerland AG 2019   119
J. D. Feuerstein, A. S. Cheifetz (eds.), *Cancer Screening in Inflammatory Bowel Disease*, https://doi.org/10.1007/978-3-030-15301-4_10

biologics in pediatric IBD is increasing [2]. Cancer risk attributed to therapy remains a controversial and emotionally charged discussion. Conflicting data regarding the risks of cancer with immunomodulators versus biologics, which is discussed in detail below, adds to the difficulty. The difficulty of investigating such an uncommon event creates uncertainty when reviewing the topic of cancer in pediatric IBD. In fact, some physicians and parents have stopped utilizing immunomodulators – citing the risk of lymphoma, personal experience of patients developing lymphoma, and, more recently, the question of their efficacy in the pediatric population. It is important to understand the evidence regarding the risk of cancer for physicians to present an unbiased appraisal of the best therapy available for each patient.

Epidemiology of Cancer in Patients with Pediatric-Onset IBD

Although the body of literature remains small, research on cancer epidemiology in pediatric IBD has expanded in the last few years. Several recent studies have investigated the overall risk of *all* forms of cancer in pediatric IBD patients and support a standardized incidence ratio (SIR) of 2.23 (95% CI: 1.98–2.52) [3–6]. A recent systematic review in 2018 by Aardoom et al. investigated the literature of all pediatric IBD patients who developed cancer. Of the 98 articles reviewed, 180 pediatric IBD patients developed cancer though it wasn't clear how many patients in total were included. The number and type of cancer included lymphoma ($n = 53$), leukemia ($n = 18$), intestinal ($n = 53$), liver ($n = 31$), skin ($n = 8$), cervical ($n = 1$), and others ($n = 16$). There were 77 fatalities related to cancer with intestinal carcinoma ($n = 34$) and lymphoma ($n = 24$) associated with the highest number of deaths [3]. Patients diagnosed with lymphoma or leukemia had a median age of 16.0 and 15.5 years old, respectively. Intestinal carcinoma occurred at a median age of 24.0 years old (range, 13.0–69.0) which was on average 11.5 years after their diagnosis with IBD. Fatal cancer outcomes occurred at the median age of 18.0 years for lymphoma and leukemia versus 25.5 for intestinal carcinoma. Overall this study found a short cancer duration before death: the median duration from cancer diagnosis to death was 1 year for 20 patients and 2 years for an addition 14 patients (Fig. 10.1) [3].

Hematologic Malignancies

Blood malignancies are the most prevalent cancers in pediatric IBD and consist of lymphoma and leukemia. In 2014, de Ridder et al. reported that 9 out of 18 pediatric IBD patients diagnosed with cancer had lymphoma [7]. A search of the United States Food and Drug Administration's (FDA) Adverse Event Reporting System (AERS) showed 15 of the 24 reported malignancies in pediatric IBD patients were lymphoma [8]. Similarly, results from a multicenter, prospective, long-term,

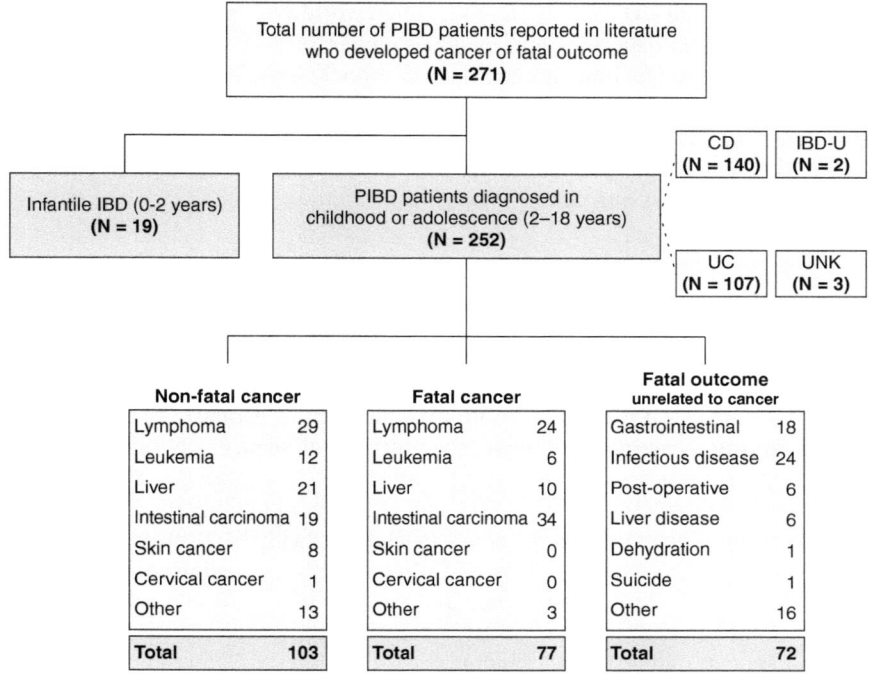

Fig. 10.1 Cancer outcomes in pediatric IBD. *CD* Crohn's disease, *UC* ulcerative colitis, *IBD-U* IBD-unclassified, *UNK* unknown. (Adapted from Aardoom et al. [3])

observational registry of pediatric patients with IBD (The DEVELOP Study) found 8 of 15 patients had either leukemia ($n = 3$) or lymphoma ($n = 5$) [4].

Hepatosplenic T-cell lymphoma (HSTCL) is an exceedingly rare and particularly deadly form of lymphoma that has been associated with IBD therapy. It has been difficult to determine the risk of HSTCL in IBD patients both due to the small number of cases and the fact that it does not typically occur during clinical trials. Post-marketing surveillance, however, has identified several patients with HSTCL. As a result, anti-tumor necrosis factor alpha (TNF) therapies and thiopurines have a warning regarding the increased risk of HSTCL in addition to lymphoma. Kotlyar et al. found 36 cases of HSTCL in patients with IBD during their review of the AERS database, 20 patients received combination therapy with azathioprine/6-mercaptopurine (AZA/6-MP) in addition to an anti-TNF and 16 patients were on monotherapy with AZA/6-MP. Interestingly, in these two groups, Crohn's patients made up 85% and 56% of cases, respectively, compared to UC patients who made up only 15% and 37.5% of the cohort. In agreement with previous reports, cases occurred predominantly in young (23 and 22.5 years old, respectively) men (male/female ratio 19:1 and 10:1, respectively, with 5 unknown) [9]. A systematic review utilized three causality assessment tools to evaluate the relationship between Crohn's disease medications and HSTCL. Thirty-seven unique and nine possible cases of HSTCL in CD patients were identified worldwide between 1998 and 2010. Unfortunately, the data does not elucidate a clear causative factor; all classes of medication (biologics, immunomodulators, aminosalicylates, steroids, and others) had a "possible" causal relationship, as the analysis was limited by the heterogeneity of case reports [10]. It is important to remind patients and their families that the risk of this malignancy is exceedingly low, even on immunomodulator therapy, as described later in this chapter.

Intestinal Malignancies

Intestinal carcinoma, colorectal carcinoma (CRC), and small bowel carcinoma closely follow blood malignancies in predominance in pediatric IBD. In fact, the risk of intestinal carcinoma is higher than blood malignancies, but is not typically diagnosed in the pediatric age group. Aardoom et al. reported a SIR of 54.7 in ulcerative colitis (UC) (95% CI: 26.0–115.4) and 6.3 in CD (95% CI: 3.93–10.2) [3]. Similarly, a Swedish cohort study of children with IBD found 122 cases of CRC during 148,682 patient years of follow-up, corresponding to a hazard ratio (HR) of 18 (14.4–22.7) when compared to healthy controls [5]. Concerningly, intestinal carcinoma is the most frequent fatal cancer in pediatric IBD. The median age of diagnosis of intestinal carcinoma was 24.0 years (16.0–69.0) with the median age of death related to intestinal carcinoma of 25.5 years (IQR = 20.0–30.5) [3]. Unlike in adult UC patients, where the risk of CRC appears to be approaching the unaffected patient risk, pediatric-onset UC continues to represent a group with increased risk [11].

Hepatic Malignancies

Liver cancer was the third most common malignancy in children with IBD, typically presenting as cholangiocarcinoma (24) and hepatocellular carcinoma (6). Interestingly, cholangiocarcinoma was fatal in only 8 of the 24 cases [3], seemingly at odds with the fulminant nature of the diagnosis in adults [12]. The large majority or risk for these liver cancers is related to patients whose UC is complicated by PSC, which is discussed later.

Dermatologic Malignancies

The role of IBD and its treatment on risk of skin cancer in pediatric IBD is not well characterized. In adults, a recent systematic review and meta-analysis in 2014 found an increased relative risk (RR) of melanoma of 1.37, which was similar between Crohn's and UC patients [13]. Similarly, adult IBD patients receiving thiopurines had a twofold higher risk of nonmelanoma skin cancer (NMSC). The risk of NMSC in patients not receiving thiopurines is unknown [14]. The risk of melanoma and nonmelanoma skin cancer in pediatric IBD patients has not been described, but health maintenance discussions should include the use of sunscreen and sun protection clothing as well as dermatologic evaluation when indicated.

Risk Factors for Malignancy in Pediatric IBD

The most obvious and important risk factor in pediatric patients with IBD is the age of onset. Patients face decades of exposure to intestinal inflammation and therapies which are at the center of the pathogenesis behind the development of cancer [15]. Pediatric IBD is also characterized by complicated disease with greater severity, extent, and more frequent use of immunomodulators and/or biologic therapies [16–18]. All of these factors are individually associated with increased cancer risk, in particular CRC and hematological malignancies. Given that cancer in pediatric IBD patients remains rare, it is difficult to characterize, as much of the knowledge regarding risk factors is extrapolated from adult studies.

Age of Onset

The age of onset of IBD has been implicated as a risk factor for CRC. A study published in *The New England Journal of Medicine* in 1990 showed patients diagnosed with pancolitis before the age of 15 years had a cumulative incidence of CRC of 40% after 35 years of disease [19]. This finding was sobering as it was much higher than previously reported. Due to the increased use of chronic therapy, the advent of biologics, and the adoption of therapeutic targets such as mucosal healing, this incidence is likely an overestimate for patients today [20]. CRC was more common in children who have ulcerative pancolitis and Crohn's patients with colonic involvement [17]. Pancolitis in UC was found to carry a relative risk of 14.8 (11.4–18.9) in a study that investigated the influence of age of onset and extent of disease on CRC risk [19]. The excess risk of CRC in Crohn's disease appears attributed to colonic involvement without an increase in relative risk in patients with only terminal ileal involvement [21].

Family History

Not to be overlooked, a family history of CRC increases risk in IBD patients, in a similar manner that it increases risk in healthy patients [22]. Clearly, if the recommendation to screen for CRC based on familial risk precedes the screening guidelines for IBD, the earlier recommendation should be followed.

Concomitant Therapies

The influence of medical therapy on cancer risk in pediatric IBD remains controversial. Initial concern regarding cancer and therapy was related to an increased risk of lymphoma [23] and nonmelanoma skin cancer [24] in adult organ transplant recipients on immunosuppressive therapies, such as thiopurines. The risk in children treated with immunomodulators appears similar to adults [25]. A meta-analysis that included 18 studies demonstrated an overall SIR for the development of lymphoma in patients receiving thiopurines for IBD of 4.92 (95% CI: 3.10–7.78). The risk of lymphoma was not significantly different in females versus males, with the exception of HSTCL where 93.5% of cases were seen in males. Patients on thiopurines for less than 1 year did not have a higher incidence of lymphoma. The largest increase in incidence occurred in patients receiving thiopurines for greater than 3 years (4.84). There was not increased incidence in patients who had received thiopurines in the past compared to patients who had never received a thiopurine. This indicates that thiopurine exposure contributes a significant risk of lymphoma in IBD patients. The risk does not appear increased if the medications are used for less than 1 year. There remains a grey zone of attributable risk for patients treated for 2–3 years. Furthermore, once thiopurines are discontinued, the risk of lymphoma eventually returns to baseline [26]. It is important to note that despite the increase in lymphoma risk with thiopurines, the absolute risk of lymphoma remains low. The incidence of lymphoma in pediatric patients is 0.58 per 10,000; thiopurine exposure increases this to 4 per 10,000 [27]. The absolute risk to pediatric IBD patients on immunomodulators for HSTCL is not known. In adult studies, the absolute risk of HSTCL is 1:45,000 for all patients on thiopurines and 1:22,000 for all patients receiving the combination of thiopurine and anti-TNF. In men younger than age 35, these risks increase to 1:7404 [28] and 1:3534, respectively [9]. Despite these low absolute risks, some physicians and patients have stopped using immunomodulators, due in part to this concern. Siegel and others have published several useful articles and tools, for assessing risk discussing it with patients and families [29–31].

Immunomodulators have also been implicated to increase the risk of nonmelanoma skin cancer in pediatric IBD patients. However, data is limited to studies in adults. A large cohort study from France reported a SIR of 2.89 (95% CI: 1.98–4.08) in all adult IBD patients and 7.06 (95% CI: 4.18–11.16) in ongoing thiopurine use versus 5.19 (95% CI: 2.37–9.86) in discontinued thiopurine use. Patients who had not received thiopurines had a SIR of 0.73 (95% CI: 0.24–1.72), suggesting the risk of NMSC is related to thiopurine use. Unlike the risk of lymphoma decreasing after discontinuation of thiopurines, the risk persists despite discontinuation of thiopurines [32]. Methotrexate is another immunomodulator used for the treatment of pediatric IBD; however its role contributing risk of cancer has not been established [33].

Understanding the risk cancer in pediatric patients receiving the various biologic therapies continues to evolve, especially given that many patients were also receiving concomitant therapy with thiopurines. Concern regarding increased risk of cancer in pediatric IBD patients receiving infliximab was initially discovered by a search of the FDA's Adverse Event Reporting System. This showed 48 reports of blood malignancy in pediatric IBD patients on either infliximab ($n = 31$), etanercept ($n = 15$), or adalimumab ($n = 2$). However, 88% of cases involved the concomitant use of other immunosuppressants (such as azathioprine, 6-mercaptopurine, and steroids) [8]. Subsequent studies have investigated whether it is the biologic therapy or the immunomodulator conferring risk. Data from the DEVELOP Registry, a multi-center prospective cohort study, and the Surveillance, Epidemiology, and End Results (SEER) database of cancer statistics in the United States, were used to determine standardized incidence ratios for malignancy in pediatric patients receiving biologics and/or immunomodulators. Patients treated with a biologic but without exposure to thiopurine had a SIR similar to the reference population: 1.11 (95% CI: 0.03–6.16). Thiopurine exposed with or without biologic treatment had a SIR of 2.88 (95% CI: 1.44–5.14). These results suggest the risk of malignancy is attributable to thiopurine exposure and that biologic use does not increase risk. However this study, as with all studies on the topic, is limited by the very low incidence of pediatric cancer in the IBD population [4]. There is also concern that anti-TNF therapy increases the risk of nonmelanoma skin cancers, as evidenced by the increased risk seen in patients with rheumatoid arthritis treated with anti-TNF agents [34]. However, this has not been confirmed in adult IBD, let alone pediatric IBD patients.

Specific cancer risk due to newer biologics such as vedolizumab (a gut-specific anti-integrin against $\alpha_4\beta_7$) and ustekinumab (an anti-IL12 and IL-23 antibody) is under investigation [35]. The concern regarding progressive multifocal leukoencephalopathy with vedolizumab treatment has dissipated with the absence of any case reports [36] but remains a concern in patients receiving natalizumab, an anti-integrin that prevents trafficking of inflammatory cells and crosses the blood-brain barrier [37].

Comorbid Conditions

One of the biggest risk factors for the development of CRC in adult IBD patients is the presence of primary sclerosing cholangitis (PSC). PSC is rare in pediatric IBD, and the literature regarding the natural history of PSC is sparse, as is the influence PSC has on pediatric cancer risk. Data extrapolated from adults suggests that pediatric PSC-IBD patients are at increased risk for CRC. A recent meta-analysis, which included 13,379 IBD patients with 1022 IBD-PSC patients, compared the risk of CRC in IBD patients with or without PSC and demonstrated an OR of 3.41 (95% CI: 2.13–5.48) [38]. Despite this extrapolation, there are no surveillance guidelines specific to pediatric PSC-IBD patients (see Surveillance section). The exact mechanism underlying the increased risk from PSC is unknown. Several hypotheses include secondary bile acids [39], Farnesoid X receptor pathway inactivation [40], and uncontrolled intestinal inflammation [41]. Persistent intestinal inflammation seems a likely mechanism. Similar to adults, pediatric IBD patients with PSC frequently have subclinical inflammation that is more likely to be extensive [42]. This was illustrated by a prospective study of 87 pediatric UC patients, 37 with PSC and 50 without PSC, which found significantly greater odds of active endoscopic and histologic inflammation in PSC patients [43].

Screening Recommendations and Approaches

Recommendations for screening by colonoscopy are limited in pediatric IBD. There are no published consensus guidelines from the North American Society of Pediatric Gastroenterology, Hepatology, and Nutrition (NASPGHAN). However, a report on health maintenance goals for IBD patients from NASPGHAN includes recommendations for cancer screening. For colorectal carcinoma it is recommended a colonoscopy with biopsies be performed at 1–2-year intervals after 7–10 years of disease. For patients with PSC, it is recommended to start screening at the time of diagnosis [44]. In pediatric patients, the recommendation is to screen every 1-2 years regardless of the exam findings, while in adults the screening can be deferred 1-3 years if the patient has two prior negative examaminations until the disease has been present for 20 years [45]. Guidelines for adults recommend screening colonoscopy with biopsies 8–10 years after diagnosis [46]. In contrast to recommendations for adults which include screening modality, there is recommendation or consensus for CRC screening modality in pediatric IBD. The benefit of high-definition endoscopy (HDE) or chromoendoscopy (CE) over white light endoscopy (WLE) in pediatrics has not been studied. The typical method is to take 4 quadrant, random, biopsies every 10 cm to have a minimum of 32 biopsies [47]. A recent adult clinical trial from Japan, found that targeted biopsies and random biopsies were able to detect similar rates of neoplasias, however, colonoscopy with targeted biopies were more cost-effective. Areas randomly biopsied without any past or present inflammation were not found to have neoplasia [48]. However, the targeted biopsy approach has not been incorporated into pediatric screening recommendations. Other forms of CRC screening in healthy adults are beginning to be explored in adult IBD patients. Areas of particular interest include stool DNA-based tests, which have demonstrated some positive results in small case series [49]. The idea to use stool tests to target endoscopic surveillance would help alleviate cost and invasive procedures [50]. Once again, this has not been evaluated in the pediatric age group.

Surveillance for other cancers associated with IBD and its therapy are even more sparse. Screening for lymphoma is by history and intermittent lab evaluation. A skin exam is recommended at each IBD visit, as is sun protection, but formal recommendations to see dermatology on a regular basis are lacking [44]. Due to the rarity of the cancer, it is probably not a cost-effective approach to broadly recommend, but it may be useful in select patients with other risk factors.

Treatment and Modifications to Therapy

The treatment of cancer in the setting of Crohn's disease and ulcerative colitis is often complicated as there are several concerns that arise. First, should the medications for IBD be continued in patients with cancer? Second, will discontinuing the medications increase the risk of flare? And third, how will therapies for IBD impact the risk of developing a second malignancy. More recently studies in the oncology literature have begun to examine the safety of specific monoclonal antibodies (MABs) for cancer in patients who have underlying IBD [51]. Clearly more research is needed as there are now numerous MABs with different mechanisms of action that are available to treat a wide variety of malignancies.

Unfortunately there are no specific treatment guidelines for the management of pediatric or adult patients with IBD and a history of malignancy. However, in 2015 the European Crohn's and Colitis Organization (ECCO) published the European Evidence-based Consensus: Inflammatory Bowel Disease and Malignancies that summarized the existing literature and provided the best guidance to date. They made several conclusions. First, based on preliminary data, anti-TNF therapy was not associated with an excess risk of developing a second cancer. Second, thiopurines, calcineurin inhibitors, and anti-TNF agents should be stopped at least until cancer therapy is complete. However, in patients with IBD and a history of malignancy, 5-aminosalicylates, nutritional therapy, and local corticosteroids can be safely used. Furthermore, they note in more severe cases not responsive to these treatments, anti-TNFs, methotrexate, short-term systemic corticosteroids, and/or surgery should be considered on a case-by-case basis. They recommend thiopurines be discontinued in IBD patients who develop squamous-cell carcinomas, aggressive forms of basal-cell carcinomas, and multiple synchronous or sequential lesions. Perhaps most importantly though, they concluded that due to the complexity of the situation, patients with cancer and IBD should be managed by a multidisciplinary team [52]. Although experts in the field agree with the ECCO Guidelines [53], there is still a need for consensus guidelines from American gastroenterological societies.

Conclusion

Cancer in pediatric IBD can occur as a result of disease activity or as an adverse effect of therapy. It is a rare event and cause of mortality for pediatric IBD patients. However, pediatric patients remain at high risk for the future development of cancer, particularly as they experience a prolonged course of illness compared to patients diagnosed as adults. It is important to screen this high-risk group appropriately for early identification and treatment. Consideration of screening frequency should also incorporate individual risk factors discussed in this chapter, such as family history, primary sclerosing cholangitis, duration of disease, pancolitis, and extensive disease. It is also important to continue treatment of colonic inflammation to reduce the risk of CAC and is a discussion point to use when families request discontinuing therapy in a patient with subclinical inflammation. More prospective studies in the pediatric population are needed, particularly regarding the risk of cancers due to therapy.

References

1. Abraham BP, Mehta S, El-Serag HB. Natural history of pediatric-onset inflammatory bowel disease: a systematic review. J Clin Gastroenterol. 2012;46(7):581–9.
2. Kugathasan S, et al. Prediction of complicated disease course for children newly diagnosed with Crohn's disease: a multicentre inception cohort study. Lancet. 2017;389(10080):1710–8.
3. Aardoom MA, et al. Malignancy and mortality in pediatric-onset inflammatory bowel disease: a systematic review. Inflamm Bowel Dis. 2018;24(4):732–41.
4. Hyams JS, et al. Infliximab is not associated with increased risk of malignancy or hemophagocytic lymphohistiocytosis in pediatric patients with inflammatory bowel disease. Gastroenterology. 2017;152(8):1901–1914.e3.
5. Olen O, et al. Childhood onset inflammatory bowel disease and risk of cancer: a Swedish nationwide cohort study 1964–2014. BMJ. 2017;358:j3951.
6. Peneau A, et al. Mortality and cancer in pediatric-onset inflammatory bowel disease: a population-based study. Am J Gastroenterol. 2013;108(10):1647–53.
7. de Ridder L, et al. Malignancy and mortality in pediatric patients with inflammatory bowel disease: a multinational study from the porto pediatric IBD group. Inflamm Bowel Dis. 2014;20(2):291–300.
8. Diak P, et al. Tumor necrosis factor alpha blockers and malignancy in children: forty-eight cases reported to the Food and Drug Administration. Arthritis Rheum. 2010;62(8):2517–24.
9. Kotlyar DS, et al. A systematic review of factors that contribute to hepatosplenic T-cell lymphoma in patients with inflammatory bowel disease. Clin Gastroenterol Hepatol. 2011;9(1):36–41.e1.
10. Selvaraj SA, et al. Use of case reports and the Adverse Event Reporting System in systematic reviews: overcoming barriers to assess the link between Crohn's disease medications and hepatosplenic T-cell lymphoma. Syst Rev. 2013;2:53.
11. Jess T, et al. Decreasing risk of colorectal cancer in patients with inflammatory bowel disease over 30 years. Gastroenterology. 2012;143(2):375–81.e1; quiz e13–4.
12. Mody K, et al. A SEER-based multi-ethnic picture of advanced intrahepatic cholangiocarcinoma in the United States pre- and post-the advent of gemcitabine/cisplatin. J Gastrointest Oncol. 2018;9(6):1063–73.
13. Singh S, et al. Inflammatory bowel disease is associated with an increased risk of melanoma: a systematic review and meta-analysis. Clin Gastroenterol Hepatol. 2014;12(2):210–8.
14. Ariyaratnam J, Subramanian V. Association between thiopurine use and nonmelanoma skin cancers in patients with inflammatory bowel disease: a meta-analysis. Am J Gastroenterol. 2014;109(2):163–9.
15. Olen O, et al. Increased mortality of patients with childhood-onset inflammatory bowel diseases, compared with the general population. Gastroenterology. 2018;156(3):614–22.
16. Vernier-Massouille G, et al. Natural history of pediatric Crohn's disease: a population-based cohort study. Gastroenterology. 2008;135(4):1106–13.
17. Van Limbergen J, et al. Definition of phenotypic characteristics of childhood-onset inflammatory bowel disease. Gastroenterology. 2008;135(4):1114–22.
18. Gower-Rousseau C, et al. The natural history of pediatric ulcerative colitis: a population-based cohort study. Am J Gastroenterol. 2009;104(8):2080–8.

19. Ekbom A, et al. Ulcerative colitis and colorectal cancer. A population-based study. N Engl J Med. 1990;323(18):1228–33.
20. Velayos FS, et al. Predictive and protective factors associated with colorectal cancer in ulcerative colitis: a case-control study. Gastroenterology. 2006;130(7):1941–9.
21. Ekbom A, et al. Increased risk of large-bowel cancer in Crohn's disease with colonic involvement. Lancet. 1990;336(8711):357–9.
22. Askling J, et al. Family history as a risk factor for colorectal cancer in inflammatory bowel disease. Gastroenterology. 2001;120(6):1356–62.
23. Kinlen LJ, et al. Collaborative United Kingdom-Australasian study of cancer in patients treated with immunosuppressive drugs. Br Med J. 1979;2(6203):1461–6.
24. Maddox JS, Soltani K. Risk of nonmelanoma skin cancer with azathioprine use. Inflamm Bowel Dis. 2008;14(10):1425–31.
25. Ashworth LA, et al. Lymphoma risk in children and young adults with inflammatory bowel disease: analysis of a large single-center cohort. Inflamm Bowel Dis. 2012;18(5):838–43.
26. Kotlyar DS, et al. Risk of lymphoma in patients with inflammatory bowel disease treated with azathioprine and 6-mercaptopurine: a meta-analysis. Clin Gastroenterol Hepatol. 2015;13(5):847–58.e4; quiz e48–50.
27. Dulai PS, Siegel CA, Dubinsky MC. Balancing and communicating the risks and benefits of biologics in pediatric inflammatory bowel disease. Inflamm Bowel Dis. 2013;19(13):2927–36.
28. Kotlyar DS, et al. Hepatosplenic T-cell lymphoma in inflammatory bowel disease: a possible thiopurine-induced chromosomal abnormality. Am J Gastroenterol. 2010;105(10):2299–301.
29. Siegel CA, et al. Real-time tool to display the predicted disease course and treatment response for children with Crohn's disease. Inflamm Bowel Dis. 2011;17(1):30–8.
30. Dubinsky MC, et al. Multidimensional prognostic risk assessment identifies association between IL12B variation and surgery in Crohn's disease. Inflamm Bowel Dis. 2013;19(8):1662–70.
31. Guizzetti L, et al. Development of clinical prediction models for surgery and complications in Crohn's disease. J Crohns Colitis. 2018;12(2):167–77.
32. Peyrin-Biroulet L, et al. Increased risk for nonmelanoma skin cancers in patients who receive thiopurines for inflammatory bowel disease. Gastroenterology. 2011;141(5):1621–28.e1–5.
33. Colman RJ, et al. Methotrexate for the treatment of pediatric Crohn's disease: a systematic review and meta-analysis. Inflamm Bowel Dis. 2018;24(10):2135–41.
34. Bongartz T, et al. Anti-TNF antibody therapy in rheumatoid arthritis and the risk of serious infections and malignancies: systematic review and meta-analysis of rare harmful effects in randomized controlled trials. JAMA. 2006;295(19):2275–85.
35. Papp K, et al. Safety surveillance for ustekinumab and other psoriasis treatments from the Psoriasis Longitudinal Assessment and Registry (PSOLAR). J Drugs Dermatol. 2015;14(7):706–14.
36. Bye WA, Jairath V, Travis SPL. Systematic review: the safety of vedolizumab for the treatment of inflammatory bowel disease. Aliment Pharmacol Ther. 2017;46(1):3–15.
37. Polman CH, et al. A randomized, placebo-controlled trial of natalizumab for relapsing multiple sclerosis. N Engl J Med. 2006;354(9):899–910.
38. Zheng HH, Jiang XL. Increased risk of colorectal neoplasia in patients with primary sclerosing cholangitis and inflammatory bowel disease: a meta-analysis of 16 observational studies. Eur J Gastroenterol Hepatol. 2016;28(4):383–90.
39. Bernstein H, et al. Bile acids as carcinogens in human gastrointestinal cancers. Mutat Res. 2005;589(1):47–65.
40. Torres J, et al. Farnesoid X receptor expression is decreased in colonic mucosa of patients with primary sclerosing cholangitis and colitis-associated neoplasia. Inflamm Bowel Dis. 2013;19(2):275–82.
41. Rubin DT, et al. Inflammation is an independent risk factor for colonic neoplasia in patients with ulcerative colitis: a case-control study. Clin Gastroenterol Hepatol. 2013;11(12):1601–8. e1–4.

42. Ricciuto A, Kamath BM, Griffiths AM. The IBD and PSC phenotypes of PSC-IBD. Curr Gastroenterol Rep. 2018;20(4):16.
43. Ricciuto A, et al. Symptoms do not correlate with findings from colonoscopy in children with inflammatory bowel disease and primary sclerosing cholangitis. Clin Gastroenterol Hepatol. 2018;16(7):1098–1105.e1.
44. Rufo PA, et al. Health supervision in the management of children and adolescents with IBD: NASPGHAN recommendations. J Pediatr Gastroenterol Nutr. 2012;55(1):93–108.
45. Itzkowitz SH, Present DH. Consensus conference: colorectal cancer screening and surveillance in inflammatory bowel disease. Inflamm Bowel Dis. 2005;11(3):314–21.
46. Huguet JM, et al. Endoscopic recommendations for colorectal cancer screening and surveillance in patients with inflammatory bowel disease: review of general recommendations. World J Gastrointest Endosc. 2017;9(6):255–62.
47. Woolrich AJ, DaSilva MD, Korelitz BI. Surveillance in the routine management of ulcerative colitis: the predictive value of low-grade dysplasia. Gastroenterology. 1992;103(2):431–8.
48. Watanabe T, et al. Comparison of targeted vs random biopsies for surveillance of ulcerative colitis-associated colorectal cancer. Gastroenterology. 2016;151(6):1122–30.
49. Johnson DH, et al. DNA methylation and mutation of small colonic neoplasms in ulcerative colitis and Crohn's colitis: implications for surveillance. Inflamm Bowel Dis. 2016;22(7):1559–67.
50. Stidham RW, Higgins PDR. Colorectal cancer in inflammatory bowel disease. Clin Colon Rectal Surg. 2018;31(3):168–78.
51. Gomez RGH, et al. Safety of bevacizumab in cancer patients with inflammatory bowel disease. J Clin Oncol. 2019;37(4_suppl):664–664.
52. Annese V, et al. European evidence-based consensus: inflammatory bowel disease and malignancies. J Crohns Colitis. 2015;9(11):945–65.
53. Kalman RS, Hartshorn K, Farraye FA. Does a personal or family history of malignancy preclude the use of immunomodulators and biologics in IBD. Inflamm Bowel Dis. 2015;21(2):428–35.

Chapter 11
Colorectal Cancer Risk and Screening in Geriatric Patients

Elissa Lin and Seymour Katz

Epidemiology of Colorectal Cancer in Elderly IBD Patients

Colorectal cancer (CRC) is the fourth most common type of cancer diagnosed in the United States behind breast, lung, and prostate cancers [1, 2]. CRC is the second leading cause of cancer-related deaths in USA for men and women combined. In 2015, there was an estimate of 1.3 million people living with CRC in the United States. The estimated number of new cases in 2018 is approximately 140,000 (both colon and rectal cancer) which represents 8.1% of all new cancer cases. The estimated number of deaths is 50,630 or 8.3% of all cancer deaths. Age plays an important role in the incidence of CRC in the United States (see Fig. 11.1). The rate of CRC in those under 65 years old is 18.2/100,000, whereas an age over 65 is associated with a rate of 185.7/100,000. Approximately 70% of cases in total develop over the age of 65, and about 40% of patients are over 75 years.

Understandably with limited life expectancy and comorbidities being more relevant, death rates also increase with age with the highest rate being 181/100,000 in the 85+ age group. Approximately 60% of cases and 70% of deaths occur in those aged 65 years and older in the United States [3]. Fortunately, when looking at the trends over the past decade (2001–2010), the overall incidence rates have decreased by an average of 3.4% per year. Among adults 50 years and older, there is a steeper decline in colorectal cancer compared to those younger than 50. This decline has been attributed to increased use of colonoscopy screening in the elderly population. However, the overall survival rate of older patients remains low. Several factors that contribute to low CRC survival rates include limited access to screening and prevalence of comorbidities which are disproportionately high in the elderly age group.

E. Lin (✉) · S. Katz
New York University Langone Health, New York, NY, USA
e-mail: elissa.lin@nyulangone.org

© Springer Nature Switzerland AG 2019

J. D. Feuerstein, A. S. Cheifetz (eds.), *Cancer Screening in Inflammatory Bowel Disease*, https://doi.org/10.1007/978-3-030-15301-4_11

131

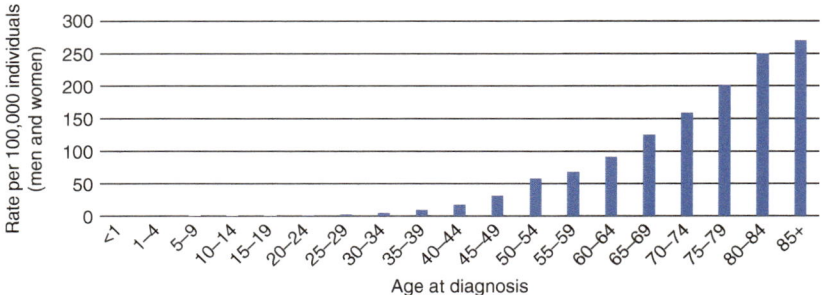

Fig. 11.1 Age-specific SEER incidence rates between 2011 and 2015 for colorectal cancer. (Adapted from *SEER Cancer Statistics Review*, 2018)

The importance of screening the elderly IBD population is highlighted by the results of a recent retrospective study which found that the incidence of CRC was significantly higher among patients who had not had a surveillance colonoscopy in the previous 36 months compared to those who had undergone the procedure (2.7% vs 1.6%) [4].

Colorectal Cancer Presentation in the Elderly

The prevalence of CRC with increasing age requires an understanding of the varied disease presentations and the biological characteristics of the cancer in the elderly and ensuring proper management. A Korean population study of over 16,000 cases found that in age groups younger than 50 and older than 50, the ascending colon was the most frequent anatomical location of colorectal polyps (40%) and adenoma was the most commonly described histology of colorectal neoplasms (CRN) [5]. In all age groups, hyperplastic polyps were mainly distributed in the distal colon and the distribution of inflammatory polyps was not significantly different among the two age groups. The major site for colorectal adenocarcinoma in both age groups was the distal colon (66.7%) except in the case of women greater than 80 years old where proximal tumor location is more likely (57%) [6].

Overall, detection rates of colorectal adenoma increase with age. The estimated risk has been shown to double from age 50–54 to age 70–74. Though sessile serrated polyps are less commonly found compared to adenomas, their prevalence increases with age [7, 8]. There is an increase in proximal tumors and decrease in rectal tumors with advancing age [6] which is important because of a higher risk of progression to cancer if polyps are found in the right versus left side of the colon [6, 9]. Additionally, right-sided CRC is associated with more methylation and microsatellite instability compared to left-sided CRC [10]. Increasing age at the time of polypectomy, in addition to polyp number, size, location, degree of dysplasia, and piecemeal resection, are associated with overall increased CRC risk [9]. Multiple studies show that older groups with CRC do not present at a more advanced stage or with worse degree of differentiation compared to their younger counterparts [11].

Predominant symptoms related to CRC in those aged 65–79 are known to be changes in stools, rectal bleeding, abdominal pain, and constipation [11]. In those ≥80 years old, the most frequent complaint is also changes in stool, followed by abdominal pain, then rectal bleeding. Older groups present with weight loss more often than those younger than 65. Perception of symptom severity and symptom disclosure is similar among all age groups. Abdominal obstruction is present in 12–18% of cases.

There are gender-specific characteristics of CRC. Increasing age in women is associated with proximal shift in CRC and it is the only independent risk factor for female CRC [6, 12]. In men, the number of concomitant adenomas significantly increases with age and it is the only independent age-related factor of male CRC [12]. Risk factors for adenoma detection include male gender and diabetes [5, 7, 8]. Age greater than 75 and male sex are also associated with an increased risk of recurrence despite stage of cancer [13].

Contributing Factors to Colorectal Cancer in the Elderly

It is estimated that 20% of CRC cases involve a family history of CRC, but the majority of CRC cases are linked to environmental factors [14]. There have been hypotheses that the increasing incidence of CRC with age is due to incremental accretion of genetic events in aging tissues; however, there has been little evidence to prove this theory. Instead, multiple molecular pathways contribute to CRC involving genetic mutations and epigenetic alterations. For example, depletion of the overall 5-methyl cytosine content occurring with age is recognized as part of the process of CRC carcinogenesis. Almost all colorectal cancers have aberrantly methylated genes particularly tumor suppressors and oncogenes.

In predictive studies of CRC risk factors, the two strongest risk factors are smoking and number of family members with CRC. The odds ratio associated with smoking is 1.75, while the odds ratio for a positive family history of CRC is 1.55 per additional family member [15]. High calcium intake has a small protective effect in patients with no previously known neoplasia. There is conflicting data regarding consumption of meat in association with detection of advanced neoplasia. Obesity in the elderly and being obese at age 21 are associated with increased risk of colorectal adenocarcinoma (CAN) [16]. Weight gain from age 18 or 10 years prior to screening is associated with a twofold increased risk of colon adenomas. Having a stably high-risk waist circumference (≥35 in. for females and ≥40 in. for males) since early adulthood is associated with a twofold increased risk of CAN. These risk factor associations may be useful in targeting select patients of the elderly population for screening.

Colorectal Cancer Risk and Presentation in Elderly Patients with Inflammatory Bowel Disease

Individuals over the age of 60 contribute to 10–15% of IBD diagnoses [17]. With an increasing population of elderly, the number of IBD patients at an advanced age is also expected to increase. Within the elderly population, however, there is a decreasing incidence of IBD with age; for example, 65% of elderly patients are aged 60–70, 25% aged 70–80, and 10% over 80 years old. Compared with younger patients, elderly patients with IBD tend to be hospitalized more given that they are more likely to be ill, malnourished, anemic, dehydrated, and hypercoagulable. The impact of cancer on the elderly may also differ given specific geriatric conditions such as comorbidities, cognition, physical impairment, and polypharmacy.

Elderly IBD patients who either have been diagnosed later in life or have had IBD for several decades present with unique features that make management of CRC risk challenging. Many questions remain as data for this elderly age group is scarce at the population level and data from clinical trials cannot be extrapolated to the elderly population as older patients are often excluded. Factors such as misdiagnosis, treatment of comorbidities, drug interactions, frailty, and social circumstances contribute to the complexities of managing the elderly patient.

Understanding CRC presentation in the elderly IBD patient is important because of the differences in clinical presentation between elderly and younger age groups. In Crohn's disease, some researchers have suggested that clinical symptoms on diagnosis are not obvious [18]. The proportion of patients with colonic involvement seems to increase with age at diagnosis which may explain how elderly patients are more likely to present with diarrhea and bleeding. The stricturing and penetrating patterns of CD are less common in patients >60 years old, whereas inflammatory disease is the predominant CD phenotype. For ulcerative colitis, the clinical course is more favorable or at least similar between elderly and younger patients and clinical symptoms on diagnosis may be more subtle in the elderly. Proctitis and left-sided UC are more common in patients >60 years than in younger patients. Location tends to remain stable with only 15% of elderly patients showing progression over time whereas the pediatric population demonstrates a 50% rate of extension. While initial attacks and relapses may be less common in the elderly population, their occurrence may be more severe.

In a multicenter case-control study evaluating the phenotype of elderly-onset IBD, authors found a lower proportion of extensive disease among elderly-onset UC patients (33% vs 39%) and an increased rate of stenosing pattern (24% vs 13%) and exclusive colonic location (28% vs 16%) in elderly-onset CD patients [19]. An older age of onset has a lower risk for CRC compared to those diagnosed with IBD at ≤15–20 years old [20, 21]. There are several explanations for this finding. For one, studies examining UC in the elderly population may exclude those who have already developed CRC or have undergone colectomy. Additionally, age of onset is an important factor as elderly-onset UC is associated with a milder and more limited disease thus reducing the risk for CRC.

Inflammatory bowel disease (IBD) is ranked among the top high-risk conditions for CRC along with familial adenomatous polyposis and hereditary nonpolyposis colorectal cancer syndrome [22]. CRC accounts for 10–15% of all deaths in IBD [23]. Approximately 18% of CRC in IBD develops within 8 years from IBD diagnosis [4]. In studies and meta-analyses, the risk of CRC in the IBD population increases with increasing disease severity, extent, and duration [20–22, 24] though there is still uncertainty as to the true degree of CRC risk for each risk factor. A 2016 population study of nearly 40,000 subjects found that the hazard ratio for developing incidental intestinal cancer in the setting of IBD was 1.42 (CI 0.99–2.06), thus suggesting only a borderline increase in risk compared to IBD-free patients [21].

In CD, the risk for CRC is increased when >30–50% of colonic mucosa is involved and in UC, there is a 10–15-fold increased risk with pancolitis and a twofold increased risk with left-sided colitis [20]. Current guidelines suggest assessing the severity of inflammation using the most recent colonoscopy alone. A recent UK study explored inflammatory burden and found that the accumulative inflammatory burden was strongly associated with CRN. This was a twofold increase in risk at approximately 10, 5, or 3.3 years of continuously mild, moderate, or severe active microscopic inflammation [25]. Thus, CRN risk stratification should involve assessment of multiple surveillance episodes.

While older age may carry an overall lower risk of CRC development compared to younger age of IBD diagnosis, CRC may develop more rapidly in elderly-onset IBD and come with other unique characteristics compared with the younger age population [26]. See Table 11.5 in the Appendix for a summary of risk factors for CRC in the patient with IBD. There is evidence that older-onset IBD patients are at increased risk for developing flat dysplasia and CRC before 8–10 years from the time of IBD diagnosis, the suggested screening guideline initiation time point. A more rapid onset of CRC in the elderly may also exist because diagnostic delay is more common in elderly than in younger IBD patients [18]. Reasons for this include a higher prevalence of IBD-like conditions such as diverticular disease and ischemic colitis that make diagnosis of IBD more difficult.

50–80% of individuals with primary sclerosing cholangitis (PSC) are later diagnosed with IBD, resulting in a phenotype that is distinct from IBD alone; this phenotype is characterized by an increased risk of CRC, extensive colitis, but mild clinical course [27]. Notably, only 0.8–5.6% of UC patients and 0.4–6.4% of CD patients will develop PSC. Neoplasia in PSC patients with colitis is more likely to occur in the proximal colon as 60% of lesions located proximal to the splenic flexure [28]. The rate of CRC multi-focality is similar in patients regardless of association with PSC [29]. The unique histomorphological features of CRC in IBD patients with and without PSC include intra-tumor lymphocytosis, Crohn's-like lymphoid reaction, mucinous features, tumor heterogeneity, well-differentiation, and lack of tumor necrosis.

The odds of CRN are more than threefold higher in those with PSC compared to IBD alone [27]. In the elderly patient with history of a quiescent, subclinical course of IBD, it is important to note that long duration of IBD is a risk factor for CRN in PSC [28]. The risk of CRN in CD patients with PSC is less known. Thus far, several single-center retrospective studies have demonstrated conflicting results, and thus further prospective cohort studies are needed to quantify the risk of CRC in CC with PSC [30]. In a Danish population-based cohort study from 1977 to 2011, results showed that PSC-IBD patients primarily had ulcerative colitis (72%), the median age at IBD diagnosis was 23 years, and the median age at PSC diagnosis was 35 years [31]. Overall survival of PSC-IBD is significantly reduced; there is a four-fold increased risk of mortality in PSC-IBD patients compared to non-PSC-IBD patients. The study showed a 20-year cumulative risk of CRC of 9% after diagnosis of both IBD and PSC which emphasizes the importance of regular colonoscopy surveillance, especially from the time of newly diagnosed PSC. Special considerations for screening and its sequelae in the elderly patient include the risk of hepatic decompensation after abdominal surgery, should a colectomy be recommended based on colonoscopy findings.

Due to the association of CRC with IBD, surveillance with screening colonoscopy should certainly be considered in the elderly population. One of the main challenges to overcome is low utilization of surveillance colonoscopy programs at the population level with only a quarter of patients undergoing surveillance at recommended intervals [20]. Even among high-risk individuals such as those with PSC, adherence to guidelines is reported to be less than 40%. The decision to pursue screening is further complicated by health-related complexities, e.g., comorbidities associated with the elderly population.

CRC Screening Modalities

The goal of screening is to reduce CRC mortality and incidence on a population basis, but there is an increasing trend toward pursuing screening on a more individualized basis. Choosing a method of screening often involves a trade-off between the degree of invasiveness of a screening test and its effectiveness in preventing cancer. Other factors to consider are the patient's willingness to undergo the test as well as degree of professional training from the provider's perspective. Optical colonoscopy (i.e., colonoscopy) is seen as the most invasive but most effective modality, while fecal occult blood testing (FOBT) is least invasive but also least effective [32]. Other screening modalities include CT colonography, Cologuard, a multi-target stool DNA test, and Epi-ProColon, a blood-based test. The concept of a screening breath test in hopes of achieving comparable sensitivity and specificity to the existing noninvasive options such as fecal immunochemical tests is under study. See Table 11.4 in the Appendix for a summary of each screening modality and their pros and cons.

Colonoscopy

Colonoscopy is considered the gold standard for CRC screening. Overall, mortality reduction with colonoscopy versus no screening ranges from 53% to 68% [5, 33]. The benefits of colonoscopy screening for CRC was demonstrated by a Veterans

Health Administration (VHA) case-control study comparing 4964 veterans with CRC age 52 and older with 19856 controls [34]. Colonoscopy reduced mortality for left-sided CRC (OR 0.28 [95% CI 0.24–0.32]) and right-sided cancer (OR 0.54 [95% CI 0.47–0.63]) to a lesser degree. Mean age was 70.8 years with a 61% reduction in CRC mortality associated with colonoscopy. The concept that colonoscopic screening extends the benefits of sigmoidoscopic screening to the entire colon has been supported by studies, although there are still some inconsistent findings regarding the degree of protection against CRC. For example, Canadian case-control studies showed a 47–67% reduction in left-sided cancer mortality with colonoscopy but no benefit in detecting proximal CRC. This is perhaps due to inexperience as non-gastroenterologists performed the procedure in most Canadian studies. In a 2018 community-based study of average-risk individuals, screening colonoscopy was associated with a 65% reduction in risk of death for right colon cancers and 75% reduction for left colon cancers compared to no screening [35]. This highlights the disparity in screening accuracy which is much dependent on various factors such as adequacy of bowel prep, diet, smoking, and operator technique and experience.

Flexible Sigmoidoscopy

While colonoscopy remains the dominant endoscopic procedure, lower GI endoscopy or flexible sigmoidoscopy is associated with a significant reduction in CRC incidence [10, 36]. However given the rightward shift in colon neoplasia with advancing age, the limited accessibility of sigmoidoscopy proximally will reduce its effectiveness in older age groups [10]. The primary mechanism by which flexible sigmoidoscopy reduces CRC-specific mortality has been shown to be mostly due to primary prevention (removal of adenomatous polyps) rather than early detection [36]. A significant disadvantage is if flexible sigmoidoscopy test results are positive, then a full colonoscopy is warranted. In the elderly population where adenomatous polyps are more prevalent than younger age groups, additional colonoscopies are more likely to be performed.

Colon Capsule Endoscopy

Colon capsule endoscopy is a minimally invasive option for assessment of the entire large bowel but still requires bowel cleansing similar to colonoscopy. It is not supported by evidence as a diagnostic modality for CRN in the surveillance of patients with inflammatory bowel disease, especially as histologic verification is required in these patients. On the other hand, the capsule may accurately assess mucosal inflammation and be useful for the assessment of mucosal change after medication changes. The concern of using the capsule in Crohn's disease is capsule retention in strictures. Studies have shown a sensitivity of 71–73% for the detection of all polyps and a specificity of 75–89% for polyps 6 mm or larger and specificity of 82–86% for more than three polyps [37]. Colon capsule endoscopy does not remove lesions and cannot be used to obtain histological samples. Studies have not validated it as a primary screening test. Instead, it is most commonly used as ancillary to the CT colonoscopy and stool DNA test.

Computed Tomography (CT) Colonography

Since its development in 1994, CT colonography has benefited from major advances including development of new-generation CT scanners, software for faster image acquisition, and better three-dimensional image quality [38]. Data from several studies show rates of detection of advanced colorectal neoplasia that range from 5.2% to 8.9% using CT colonography compared to 7.1–8.6% using optical colonoscopy. CT colonography may also be advantageous for finding adenomas located at the proximal side of haustral folds or inner curve of flexures which otherwise may be missed by colonoscopy. However, the absolute risk difference in advanced colorectal neoplasia detection was −0.02 in favor of optical colonoscopy, thus supporting optical colonoscopy as the gold standard. Randomized trials are still needed to assess the effect of CT colonography screening on CRC incidence and mortality.

Magnetic Resonance (MR) Colonography

MR colonography is an attractive option compared to CT colonography because of its lack of ionizing radiation. Due to its ability to offer excellent soft-tissue contrast, MR colonography is used for the evaluation of various abdominal abnormalities including inflammatory bowel disease. For use in CRC screening, MR colonography requires bowel preparation and distension of the colon. Potential downsides to MR colonography are false-positive filling detects caused by air or residual stool [39]. Graser et al. showed the sensitivity and specificity for detecting adenomas larger than 10 mm to be 90.9% and 98.5% respectively [40]. Data on detection rates for different morphologic features of adenomas is limited but necessary given the prevalence of flat lesions in the IBD population.

Barium Enema

The double-contrast barium enema (DCBE), also known as air-contrast barium enema or lower GI series, involves barium sulfate and air insufflated into the colon through the anus. DCBE is seen as safer and less expensive than colonoscopy and is occasionally used as a follow-up test in patients with incomplete colonoscopy where cancers in the proximal portion of the colon might have evaded visualization by endoscopy [41]. However, this screening modality has been in decline over the years. Organizations such as the U.S. Preventive Services Task Force have excluded DCBE as a screening option due to a low sensitivity of detecting polyps of 48% in multiple studies [33].

Fecal Occult Blood Test

Fecal occult blood tests include the guaiac-based FOBT and newer fecal immuno-chemical tests (FIT). These tests rely on the detection of the presence of hemoglobin in feces through a chemical reaction dependent upon the peroxidase activity of heme [33, 42]. This in turn, depends on the neoplastic lesion having a bleeding phenotype. Once-only test sensitivity for cancer is approximately 50%. In addition, FOBT can be a two-step screening process where the test selects participants at a higher risk of cancer who may proceed to colonoscopy for further diagnostic investigation. In multiple guaiac-based FOBT randomized controlled trials, the likelihood of finding a cancer given a positive test was 8-fold to 25-fold times greater relative to colonoscopy without any intervening test [42]. In a 30-year follow-up of participants randomly assigned to annual screening with FOBT vs controls, a 32% reduction in the rate of death from CRC was observed [43]. However, FOBT did not significantly reduce all-cause mortality.

Fecal Immunochemical Test

FIT has been the noninvasive test of choice in organized screening programs in Europe and is shown to be superior to FOBT in the detection of advanced adenomas. Recent data suggests that FIT every 2 years for five rounds can detect advanced neoplasia at a similar rate as a one-time colonoscopy [44]. However FIT suffers from a high variation in sensitivity (61–91%) [45] subject to the effect of seasonal variation on test performance. European and Korean studies have shown that the positivity rate of FIT is reduced in summer months (June, July, August) which is thought to be due to high ambient temperatures worsening the performance of FIT [46]. Positive predictive value and interval cancer rate was found to be higher in the summer. Cancer detection rate was similar in all seasons. Also important to note is a distinction between qualitative and quantitative FIT. Quantitative FIT has lower sensitivity than qualitative FIT (73% vs 85%) but a higher positive predictive value. Qualitative tests visually indicate when hemoglobin is detected, whereas quantitative FITs measure the amount of hemoglobin numerically and report the result as positive if greater than a pre-specified threshold.

Stool DNA Test

In a cross-sectional study of 12,776 participants that compared a multi-target stool DNA test (Cologuard) with a commercial FIT among patients at average risk for CRC, the sensitivity of the DNA test for the detection of CRC and advanced precancerous lesions exceeded that of FIT by almost 20 percentage points [47]. The DNA test was 92.3% sensitive for CRC compared to 73.8% for FIT, and 42.4% sensitive for advanced precancerous lesions compared to 23.8%. FIT-Cologuard included quantitative molecular assays for KRAS mutations, aberrant NDRG4 and BMP3 methylation, and ß-actin in addition to the hemoglobin immunoassay. Patients may prefer certain benefits of cologuard. For example, the test can be completed from home and mailed directly to a lab. Additionally, there is preservation of patient privacy, safety/no need for sedation, no need for bowel prep, and no lost time from work.

Blood Test

The Epi proColon blood test or mSEPT9 assay is an annual test that is indicated for average-risk CRC adults [32], though not recommended by the US Multi-Society Task Force on CRC [48]. It searches for aberrantly methylated genes and only requires a small sample of blood. Relative to Cologuard, the Epi proColon is less sensitive for both CRC and advanced adenomas (sensitivity 48.2% and 11.2% respectively). However, the Epi proColon has a high specificity of 91.5% for CRC. Though the Epi proColon falls short in detecting advanced adenomas, it may be an option for the frail elderly where precancerous lesions are of less clinical concern. Furthermore, new serum biomarkers for the diagnosis of colon cancer are being discovered such as COL10A1 (collagen protein expressed in cancer tissue) which attained a 63% sensitivity and 85% specificity for colon cancer or adenoma in a study involving 80 colon cancer cases, 23 patients with adenoma, and 77 cancer-free controls [49].

Breath Test

In recent decades, an increasing amount of research has been dedicated to the identification of volatile organic compounds (VOC) in various excreted biological materials. The concept centers on VOCs serving as biomarkers of disease. Using a breath, urine, blood, or fecal sample, these tests would involve complex analysis of VOC patterns that can discriminate between patients with CRC and health individuals [45, 50]. Small pilot studies have found that VOC analysis can identify CRC with a sensitivity of 30–94% and a specificity of 60–94%. Questions still remain regarding its application in clinical practice. There is still uncertainty as to whether or not VOC patterns are specific to CRC as opposed to other colonic diseases such as IBD or diverticular disease. The technique of VOC analysis is not standardized and there is debate as to which biologic sample is most advantageous for CRC screening. That said, breath testing is thought to be most convenient for the patient, least invasive, and likely the least costly. Thus far, no studies have compared a VOC breath or fecal test with FIT, but there is the potential for VOC analysis to have higher sensitivity and patient compliance compared to FIT.

Barriers to Pursuing Colonoscopy in the Elderly

Barriers to pursuing surveillance colonoscopy for the frail elderly begin with patient acceptance of the procedure and proper education of the purpose, risks, preparation, and safety measures. In a survey of 100 IBD patients, only 7% spontaneously mentioned CRC risk as a main feature of IBD and 66% of patients knew that IBD increases CRC risk [51]. Gastroenterologists were the main and preferred source of information for the majority of patients. If colectomy were to be recommended in the case of non-adenoma-like raised lesions or flat high-grade dysplasia, only 25% of patients stated they would follow this recommendation for fear of definitive ostomy or complications of surgery.

Analysis of a survey of 88 elderly patients undergoing surveillance colonoscopy showed that difficulty ambulating, difficulty performing activities of daily living, and history of diabetes were significant univariate predictors of inadequate bowel preparation though only difficulty ambulating was an independent predictor [52]. Patients who have difficulty ambulating may fear incontinence and subsequently consume a less than optimal amount of preparation solution. Factors from the patient perspective that influence patient agreement to screening include test-related embarrassment and fear of pain [53]. Alternatively, patients are more willing to accept screening if offered an interview with a health professional or offered a non-invasive test alternative.

With regards to sedation, in the past, midazolam, fentanyl, and propofol have been the most commonly used sedatives for colonoscopy [54]. In general, adverse effects of conscious sedation are uncommon. These agents provide patient comfort, reduce procedure time, and improve examination quality during colonoscopy. Choice of sedative depends on age, anxiety, comorbidities, and baseline medications. In the elderly age group, risks of sedation are complicated by increased rates of aspiration, hypoxia, arrhythmias, and hypotension. In an analysis of over 1.3 million colonoscopies performed from 2000 to 2013, the use of propofol for deep sedation has greatly increased while the use of meperidine has declined. Several studies have shown that propofol can be safely used in the elderly despite its propensity to lower blood pressure [55]. Childers et al. showed that the use of diazepam has dropped out of favor since 2003 and the average dose of medication used for individual compounds has not significantly changed over time [54]. However, the same study showed a significant age-dependent decline in the dose of sedatives (with the exception of histamine-1 receptor antagonists).

There is evidence that elderly patients require less sedation during endoscopy than younger counterparts with similar satisfaction rates and procedural outcomes [54]. This can be explained by physiologic processes occurring with age such as decreasing total body water and increasing body fat resulting in increased serum concentrations after a bolus administration of drug and greater volume of distribution prolonging drug action [56]. While sedation and analgesia for patients undergoing colonoscopy is standard practice in the U.S., unsedated colonoscopy is often performed in Asia and Europe. In a retrospective study comparing tolerance of colonoscopy with and without sedation, non-sedative colonoscopy was associated with shortened hospital stay time, improved ability to return to work earlier, and was tolerated by 91% of patients [57].

In a prospective single-center study evaluating tolerance of colonoscopy with conventional versus ultrathin colonoscopes (UTC) in ulcerative colitis patients, the flexible ultrathin colonoscope was significantly better tolerated [58]. In a recent meta-analysis that examined the performance of ultrathin colonoscopes, there was no difference in cecal intubation time between UTC and standard colonoscopes, and polyp and adenoma detection rates were similar between both devices [59]. This meta-analysis confirmed that pain scores were significantly lower with UTC. UTC can potentially decrease the need for analgesia further reducing cardiopulmonary risks associated with deep sedation. Concerns with UTC are mainly susceptibility to excessive looping which could increase risk of perforation and result in incomplete colonoscopy. Looping was found to be the leading cause of incomplete colonoscopy with UTC (1.2% of procedures) compared with standard colonoscopes (0.2%).

Adverse Events of Colonoscopy in the Elderly

The major concern for performing colonoscopy in the elderly patient is the increased risk for complications which can occur during, immediately after, or delayed (see Fig. 11.2). The overall complication rate in patients over 80 is low, ranging from 0.2% to 0.6% [55]. However, a retrospective cohort study on patients undergoing screening colonoscopy from 2001 to 2010 found that age greater than 75 years was independently associated with increased risk of hospitalization following colonoscopy (adjusted OR 1.28; 95% CI 1.07–1.53) [60]. Physiologic changes in addition to the increased development of comorbidities make the elderly population particularly complex. Age-related changes include aspiration pneumonia or pneumonitis due to declining gag reflex [61]. The elderly also have higher rates of nonsteroidal anti-inflammatory drug use and reduced mucosal protective barriers which contribute to an increased risk of gastrointestinal bleeding, especially in the setting of endoscopic procedures such as polypectomies. Increased age is also associated with a higher degree of diverticular disease which can lead to longer duration of the procedure. There is an increased risk of perforation with ever year increase in age

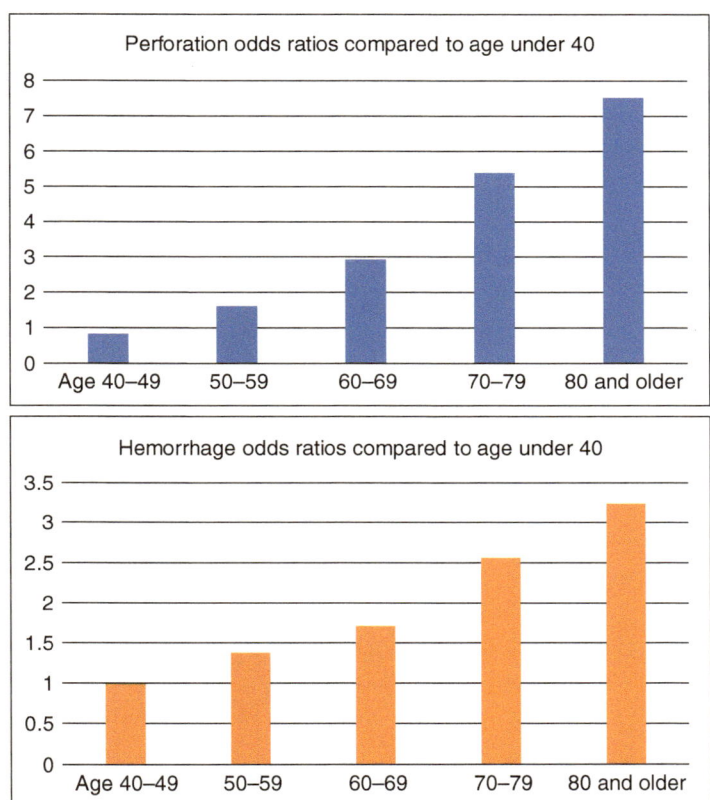

Fig. 11.2 Adverse events associated with colonoscopy by age. (Data obtained from Lin et al. [76])

adding an additional 1% risk of perforation. Those aged older than 80 have a perforation incidence of 115 per 100,000 colonoscopies.

Cardiopulmonary complications are the most common periprocedural adverse events in the elderly who are at increased risk compared to younger patients. Cardiovascular complications occur despite elderly patients on average receiving lower doses of sedatives [55]. Thirty days after colonoscopy, the risk of non-gastrointestinal/cardiopulmonary events is increased, likely due to colonoscopy exacerbating underlying comorbid illness. Post-procedural cardiopulmonary events are more likely to occur in those taking antithrombotic medications and those with pulmonary comorbidities. Post-procedural cardiopulmonary events also increase with age in patients even without comorbidities compared to average-risk patients younger than 50 [62].

In a population-based prospective study of Medicare beneficiaries ages 70–79, adverse events were compared between age groups 70–74 and 75–79 and regardless if colonoscopy was performed [63]. Overall, the excess risk of serious adverse events with colonoscopy within 30 days was small in both age groups (see Fig. 11.3).

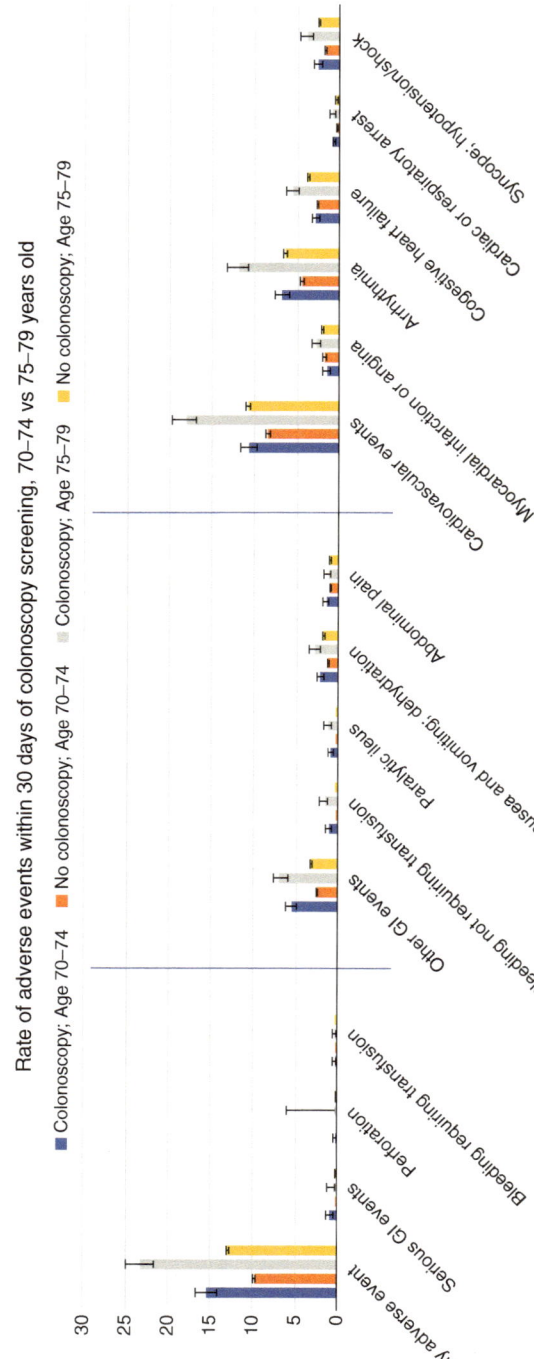

Fig. 11.3 Standardized risk per 1000 patients for adverse events within 30 days of colonoscopy screening. (Data obtained from Garcia-Albeniz et al. [63])

In both age groups, colonoscopy was associated with an excess risk of less than 2 events per 1000 patients with the exception of arrhythmias which occurred with an excess risk of 2.4 cases per 1000 individuals in the 70–74 age group and of 5.5 cases per 1000 individuals in the 75–79 age group. An increased risk of arrhythmias in the elderly can be explained by physiologic changes, such as a decreased beta-adrenergic responsiveness, increased fibrotic infiltration of cardiac conduction pathways, and an increased reliance on the Frank-Starling mechanism leading to conduction abnormalities and other cardiovascular problems [56].

Patient discomfort has been noticed to be higher in patients aged <75 (1.1% of patients) and lowest in patients >86 (0% of patients) [64]. Post-procedural self-reported symptoms over all age groups are most commonly bowel distension and abdominal pain [53]. Some patients report fecal incontinence, but overall, these symptoms are generally self-limited and last no more than a day.

Bowel Preparation in the Elderly

Adequate bowel preparation is essential for proper visualization of mucosa during colonoscopy. Inadequate bowel preparation can be a cause for an incomplete colonoscopy. In a meta-analysis of 20 studies, suboptimal bowel preparation was documented in 18.8% of patients >65 years of age and in 12.1% in patients >80 [65]. Physiologic reasons for inadequate bowel preparation in the elderly include slower colonic transit and higher incidence of obstipation.

The main components of cleansing agents are peroral polyethylene glycol (PEG) solution, sodium phosphate, or sodium sulfate. However the leading choice for bowel preparation in the elderly is polyethylene glycol which is generally well tolerated despite the large volume load (4 L). It has a lower risk of electrolyte depletion or renal injury [61, 66]. The split-dose method of giving half the bowel preparation dose on the same day as the endoscopy results in higher quality colonoscopy and increases adenoma detection rate compared to ingestion of the entire preparation the day before endoscopy [67]. This method also further reduces the risk of non-compliance, fluid shifts, and renal injury in the elderly which is more likely to occur with small volume osmotic laxatives such as sodium sulfate.

Adverse events related to bowel preparation include interactions with existing medications. Since the elderly have the highest rates of polypharmacy, it is important to look for antihypertensive and diuretic use as bowel preparation increases the risk of dehydration and periprocedural hypotension. Furthermore, the elderly are at risk for impaired thirst reflex and inadequate renal free water handling. Patients with poor renal function, dehydration, hypercalcemia, or treatment with angiotensin-converting enzyme inhibitors or angiotensin receptor blockers may experience phosphate nephropathy after the use of sodium phosphate solutions, the risk of which is increased with age [61]. Therefore, sodium phosphate is not recommended in the elderly. Adequate hydration with clear liquids up to 2 hours before endoscopy should be encouraged to avoid hypotension. For diabetes management, oral antihyperglycemics should not be taken on the morning of the procedure, and long-acting insulin formulations should be halved. Because of the risk of hypoglycemia in the elderly, early morning procedures are preferred.

From the patient perspective, bowel preparation is seen as the most burdensome aspect of CRC screening, especially given its side effects of nausea, vomiting, and abdominal pain [67]. These side effects increase with age. With this in mind, in the elderly population, it is important to assess for comorbidities, ability to consent, and ability to successfully follow pre-procedural and post-procedural instructions. A lack of understanding regarding pre-endoscopy instructions can result in unsuccessful bowel preparation and inaccurate endoscopy findings.

Colorectal Cancer Screening Strategies in the Elderly Patient with IBD

Current Screening Recommendations

Current screening guidelines do not distinguish the elderly patient with IBD from the general population except in noting that surveillance should be applied only to those whose life expectancy is expected to benefit and those who can tolerate the procedures. Patients with IBD at all ages have an overall survival that is comparable to or only slightly lower than that of the general population though age is reported as an independent risk factor for mortality among IBD patients even after adjusting for comorbidity [18].

Society guidelines generally agree on appropriate time to begin surveillance for CRC but vary on appropriate intervals between surveillance colonoscopies. There is also question as to the most appropriate methods and techniques of surveillance. In the IBD population where CRC is a well-known complication, it is crucial to understand best screening methods to prevent CRC, a likely cause of mortality. It is also important to approach the elderly population with IBD as two groups: those diagnosed at a younger age (before the age of 60) and those with onset of IBD at a later age (late-onset IBD) given that long-standing IBD confers a higher risk of CRC. Late-onset IBD is not associated with an increased risk of CRC when compared to non-IBD patients, yet elderly-onset IBD patients may develop CRC more rapidly (i.e., within 8 years) [26].

Among the various guidelines for CRC screening in the patient with IBD, surveillance imaging is not appropriate based on the American College of Radiology Appropriateness Criteria [68]. Given that patients with IBD are considered high risk for CRC, screening should be performed during clinical remission of disease in order to distinguish inflammatory changes from dysplasia [22]. The American Gastroenterological Association suggests that surveillance colonoscopy should be initiated at maximum 8 years after the onset of IBD symptoms. Various organizations differ slightly on the exact timing of the first screening and intervals. For example, the European Crohn's and Colitis Organization and the American College of Gastroenterology (ACG) suggest first time screening 8–10 years after the onset of symptoms. Regular surveillance should be continued but the interval between colonoscopies has not been standardized. The British Society of Gastroenterology differs from other societies by including risk stratification in determining surveillance intervals. CRC risk profile should be determined in the first surveillance colonoscopy. In both European and American IBD organizations, surveillance interval ranges are 1–3 years. Evidence from RCTs support that for the patient with UC and left-sided colitis or extensive colitis, screening colonoscopy be performed annually or biennially [69]. In the case of CD, patients with disease affecting more than one-third of the colon should also undergo surveillance colonoscopy annually or bienni-ally. In the elderly IBD patient with only left-sided colitis or Crohn's colitis with <50% of the colon involved, European societies recommend screening every 5 years as opposed to yearly exams [70]. Special consideration should be paid to the elderly patient with PSC as there is an elevated risk of CRC that is nearly fourfold the risk in those without PSC. Societies currently recommend annual surveillance from time of diagnosis of PSC in a patient with IBD, regardless of the subtype (See Table 11.1).

The International Agency for Research on Cancer reports sufficient evidence for CRC surveillance in the IBD population with currently established stool-based tests and lower endoscopy as these methods reduce the risk of death from CRC and ben-efits outweigh the harms [44]. Method of choice for surveillance in the elderly patient with IBD depends on multiple factors: from patient selection, to ability to perform the procedure successfully, to alignment with the elderly patient's goals of care. The mainstay of CRN detection for patients with IBD remains surveillance

Table 11.1 Summary of society guidelines for CRC surveillance in IBD patients including timing, intervals, and recommended technique [71]

Low risk (every 5 years)	Intermediate (every 3 years)	High risk (annually)
Colitis affecting <50% of the colon	Extensive colitis with mild inflammatory activity	Extensive colitis with mod/severe inflammation
Extensive colitis with no or mild endoscopic/histological inflammation	Postinflammatory polyps	Primary sclerosing cholangitis
Crohn's colitis affecting <50% of the colon	Family history of CRC in first-degree relative >50 years old	Stricture in past 5 years
UC without high-risk features on 2 previous colonoscopies	Quiescent UC without high-risk features	Dysplasia in past 5 years (no surgery)
		First-degree relative with CRC <50 years
		Chronically active UC
		Shortened colon
		Inflammatory polyps

Adapted from British Society of Gastroenterology, European Crohn's and Colitis Organization, and the Australian Cancer Council colonoscopy using white light endoscopy [4]. The aim is to detect and remove dysplastic lesions thereby preventing cancer and CRC-related mortality.

During the colonoscopy, previously established protocol was two to four random biopsies that should be taken every 10 cm along the entire colon with additional samples taken from suspicious areas. However newer more efficient strategies for detection of neoplastic lesions have been utilized. Among gastroenterologists, recent studies have shown that compliance with the recommended number of biopsies is less than 50% [4]. With the transition to high-definition (HD) endoscopes, there may not be a need for random biopsies given the ability to visualize colitis-associated CRN. Some guidelines also state that all biopsies should be taken from mucosa surrounding visibly suspected lesions in order to ensure complete removal of the lesion. However a recent study of 1065 IBD patients examining the clinical consequences of surrounding mucosal biopsies found that the dysplasia yield of surrounding mucosal biopsies was only 5% [72]. In this era of high-definition endoscopes and other imaging techniques (discussed below), the practice to routinely take surrounding mucosal biopsies may no longer be useful or cost-effective.

To further improve the diagnostic yield of biopsies, focus has been placed on endoscopic techniques such as chromoendoscopy that uses dye to detect colonic lesions to be biopsied. Based on meta-analysis including randomized controlled trials, the use of chromoendoscopy with 0.1% of indigo carmine or 0.1% of methylene blue showed a significantly higher intraepithelial neoplasia detection rate compared with white light endoscopy [69]. Total examination time is significantly shorter using targeted biopsies which may be beneficial in the elderly when duration under sedation is important. Random biopsies from areas without any signs of present or past inflammation do not typically yield neoplastic tissue. Independent predictors of dysplastic histology are location in the proximal colon, protruding morphology, loss of innominate lines, and neoplastic pit patterns [73]. ACG recommendations from 2018 state insufficient evidence for universal chromoendoscopy for IBD colorectal neoplasia surveillance and instead suggest limiting chromoendoscopy for patients at high risk [74]. Chromoendoscopy requires skilled operator dependence and need for adequate bowel preparation. A prospective trial comparing narrow-band imaging (NBI) to conventional colonoscopy and chromoendoscopy found NBI to be less time-consuming without a difference in dysplasia detection [75]. However, NBI misses suspicious lesions 30.7% more than chromoendoscopy and is therefore not considered a substitute for chromoendoscopy.

Does Colorectal Cancer Screening Extend Life in the Elderly?

From 2008 until 2018, the American Cancer Society, the US Multi-Society Task Force on Colorectal Cancer, and the American College of Radiology have stood by consensus guidelines for the detection of adenomatous polyps and CRC in average-risk adults using screening colonoscopy [2, 61, 76]. These societies do not indicate an upper age limit due to a lack of current data. The U.S. Preventive Services Task

Force and American College of Physicians recommend an upper age limit of 75 based on systematic reviews that suggest a limited benefit to routine screening beyond age 75 [61, 76]. However, this guidance is currently under review. Given that the number of individuals over age 86 is expected to double by the year 2030, there is suggestion that those between ages 75 and 85 years should be screened on an individual assessment of risk versus benefit [37].

In a 2017 network meta-analysis of screening modalities in CRC [65], the relative risk of mortality due to CRC was 0.86 for FOBT compared with no screening. FIT reduced CRC mortality by 59% and FS resulted in a 33% reduction in CRC mortality. When FS was combined with FOBT, CRC mortality was reduced by 38%. Colonoscopy resulted in 61% reduction in CRC mortality. However no randomized trials have shown a benefit in mortality. The question remains if these screening modalities are effective at extending life in the elderly when life expectancy becomes a relevant consideration.

A population-based study of Medicare beneficiaries aiming to evaluate the effectiveness of colonoscopy screening found that in the 70–74 age group, the standardized 8-year risk of CRC was 2.19% in the colonoscopy screening arm and 2.62% in the no screening arm, a risk difference of −0.42% [63]. In the 75–79 age group, the standardized 8-year risk of CRC was 2.84% in the colonoscopy screening arm and 2.97% in the no screening arm, a risk difference of −0.14%. The authors concluded that their findings were consistent with USPSTF recommendations for routine screening until age 75 followed by individualized decisions afterward. Though this study did not include CRC-specific mortality rates, the expectation is that CRC mortality and morbidity would be lower in the screening arm given the increased detection of CRC cases, the majority of which were stage 0 and I.

In a case-control study involving veterans aged 52 years or older, CRC screening was associated with less mortality reduction in right-sided CRC compared to left-sided CRC (46% vs 72% reduction in mortality) [34]. In a separate case-control study determining the association of CRC with exposure to lower GI endoscopic procedures (colonoscopy and sigmoidoscopy) in veterans age 75 and older, exposure to colonoscopy over a 10-year period was associated with a significant reduction in both distal and proximal CRC (OR 0.45 distal CRC, OR 0.67 proximal CRC) [10]. However, sigmoidoscopy over the same 10-year period was not significantly associated with reduction in either distal or proximal CRC. Thus, sigmoidoscopy may not be an effective strategy for preventing CRC in the elderly.

In the general population, modeling studies have shown that routine screening colonoscopy in the very elderly (≥80 years of age as defined by the World Health Organization) results in only a fraction of the expected life expectancy extension in younger patients [77]. One study estimated a mean extension in life expectancy in the group aged 80 years or older to be 0.13 years vs an extension of 0.85 years in the 50–54 years old group [55]. This may be due to competing risk of mortality from other comorbid diseases. A 2017 Cochrane analysis was performed to assess the effectiveness of cancer surveillance programs for the diagnosis of IBD-associated CRC and reduction of mortality rate from CRC [78]. The review found a higher rate of cancer occurred in the non-surveillance group compared to the surveillance group, the odds of CRC development were reduced by 42%, and odds of death by CRC was reduced by 64%. However, with only observational data included and no prospective data, the quality of evidence for this review was low for any survival benefit with surveillance colonoscopy. Detection of earlier stage CRC with surveillance may explain some survival benefit which may also be attributed to lead time bias, enhanced medical therapies to control inflammation, or chemoprevention with 5-aminosalicylates.

Given the intensive surveillance protocols detailed for the IBD patient with CRC risk factors, there is question as to what degree increased screening frequency contributes to reduced mortality from CRC. The Cochrane review reports weak evidence that surveillance colonoscopy prolongs survival in extensive colitis, though surveillance is likely to be effective in reducing the risk of death from colorectal adenocarcinoma [78]. In a retrospective study by Eluri et al. [79], in patients with IBD, nearly 30% of high-grade dysplasia (HGD)/CRC was found at colectomy which was missed on prior colonoscopy. All of these CRC cases had prior colonoscopies that showed either low-grade dysplasia (LGD) within a rectosigmoid stricture, multifocal polypoid LGD, or an unresectable lesion with LGD. These results emphasize the importance of aggressive surveillance, particularly in those with colonic strictures, right-sided location, and rectal areas where HGD/CRC can be easily missed. The risk of progression from LGD to HGD or CRC remains controversial as low numbers of LGD lesions that progress to HGD or CRC may be due to the improvement of therapies and surveillance strategies. Multivariate logistic regression analysis shows that the risk of early or missed CRCs is three times higher for IBD patients which further supports intensive surveillance colonoscopy for the elderly IBD patient [18].

The benefit of surveillance colonoscopy also involves consideration of the procedural yield, defined as the percentage of patients who are found to have significant findings on colonoscopy. Trends show that the yield of colonoscopy increases with age corresponding to the higher prevalence of colorectal neoplasia in the elderly [55]. Yield for colorectal neoplasia ranges from 3.7% to 14.2% in patients >65 years old. Studies evaluating patients 80 or older show that cancers are detected in 11–14% of cases and adenomas and polyps in roughly 19–30% of cases.

Deciding Whether or Not to Screen the Elderly Patient

The decision to screen in the elderly population depends on multiple variables such as CRC risk, life expectancy, risk of the screening procedure, cost-effectiveness, and ability for the elderly patient to withstand treatment should screening result in suspicious findings (see Table 11.2) [80]. Guiding all screening decisions is the principle that surveillance should be done only if patients are fit to undergo colectomy should dysplasia be found. In the IBD population, while guidelines exist regarding when to dial down aggressive screening, there have not been studies that specifically assess outcomes and recommendations in the elderly IBD patient. As

Table 11.2 Considerations for CRC screening with colonoscopy in elderly IBD patients

Patient-related	Procedure-related
Comorbidities	Sedation/anesthesia complications
Polypharmacy	Colonoscopy complications
Patient desires	Bowel prep complications and completion
Nutritional status	% yield of colonoscopy
Life expectancy	Psychosocial support
Frailty status	Patient ability to undergo chemotherapy/radiation
Cognitive impairment status	Quality of life
Access to medical care	

such, it is important to make individualized decisions in this population. Several important questions should be addressed in making the decision to screen. What is the patient's life expectancy and does colonoscopy offer a benefit? Is the patient able to tolerate the preparation and screening procedure? What is the likelihood of detecting CRN and can the patient undergo treatment?

The American College of Physicians recommends that average-risk CRC screening be discontinued in patients with a life expectancy of <10 years. Since the elderly IBD patient is at increased risk for CRC, tools that take into consideration comorbidities are useful for making screening decisions. Quantitative tools are readily available for estimating life expectancy, some even taking into consideration CRC risk. A 2011 systematic review on prognostic indices aided in the development of a tool called *ePrognosis* which is helpful for determining life expectancy in the elderly without a dominant terminal illness [81]. Screeningdecision.com is another tool that specifically assesses personalized risks and benefits of colonoscopy screening taking into consideration life expectancy. Important to note is that this model does not allow for the option to specify inflammatory bowel disease as the cause of increased risk for CRC and there is no option to set the most recent colonoscopy to less than 10 years. Presumably, those with inflammatory bowel disease can be screened more frequently.

It is important to start with a full history, since patients may not remember details of prior colonoscopies. The medical history can aid in determining the patient's ability to undergo the full colonoscopy preparation and procedure. Prior endoscopy reports may be useful in assessing procedure completion and patient tolerance. Family history and genetic risk scores can be used when stratifying CRC risk for screening. A German study involving a population of 2363 CRC patients and 2198 controls found that a CRC family history was associated in 316 cases (13.4%) versus 214 controls (9.7%, p value <0.0001) [82]. There was also a 2.9-fold (OR 2.94) increased risk of CRC with genotype adjusted for sex and age. The risk increased 1.5-fold (OR 1.47) if family history included a first-degree relative. Once hospitalized, older patients tend to be sicker, malnourished, hypovolemic, more anemic, and have increased transfusion requirements [18]. Even after adjusting for comorbidities in the IBD patient, age is predictive of in-hospital mortality.

To improve colonoscopy yield in the IBD patient, a mean severity score can be quickly calculated based on the segment worst affected by colitis seen in the preceding 5–10 years of colonoscopies [25]. Mean severity scores are significantly more accurate than maximum severity scores or findings from only the most recent colonoscopy. Patients with severe or persistent disease should be considered for more frequent surveillance and undergo active treatment.

Overall, the cost of screening increases with age, while cost-effectiveness and quality-adjusted life years (QALY) decrease. QALY is a useful measure of health outcomes that combines duration and quality of life. These trends are not affected by sex or race. Screening history and comorbidity status have an impact on the effectiveness of colonoscopy screening in the elderly. CRC risk can be calculated using the National Cancer Institute's Colorectal Cancer Risk Assessment Tool designed by health providers for patients between the ages of 50 and 85 [83].

Taking screening history and CRC risk into account, screening is cost-effective until 66 years for previously screened, low-risk individuals, whereas screening up to age 88 is cost-effective for healthy yet high-risk individuals [80]. In a retrospective study comparing data from extremely elderly patients (>90 years) to elderly patients (75–79 years), diagnostic colonoscopy was found to be associated with increased risk for incomplete procedure, inadequate bowel preparation, and adverse events mostly attributed to cardiopulmonary events [84]. However, advanced neoplasias were significantly more common in the extremely elderly group. Given that the appropriate age to stop screening varies among individuals, it is important to consider these factors to avoid harm.

In addition to analyzing the risks and benefits of screening colonoscopy, it is important that decisions are made in line with patient goals of care. In a Veterans Affairs study assessing patients' attitudes toward de-intensifying or ceasing surveillance, 51% of patients were comfortable with stopping surveillance in the setting of poor health, but comfort with the decision rose with education and trust in the physician [85]. Methods of predicting adverse events in the elderly undergoing colonoscopy are mostly based on retrospective studies; therefore, prospective studies are much needed to identify the most vulnerable elderly anticipating undergoing screening colonoscopies.

Fit Versus Frail

Selection of the appropriate CRC screening modality must include a frailty evaluation in addition to conventional CRC risk factors. Frailty defined by geriatricians is a syndrome of decreased reserve and resistance to stress resulting in a decline in multiple organ systems. Frailty is not synonymous with comorbidity or disability. Instead, comorbidity is a risk factor and disability is an outcome of frailty. There are a number of scores that quantify frailty, some of which perform better than chance at predicting adverse outcomes (see Table 11.3). There is still much need for prospective studies to identify the most vulnerable elderly anticipating screening colonoscopies.

Table 11.3 Frailty scores, advantages and disadvantages

Frailty score	Advantages	Disadvantages
Hospital Frailty Risk Score by Gilbert et al. [86]	Validated in a large English inpatient database Useful for risk stratification in emergency care settings	Classifies mortality risk moderately well Frailty among elderly with few or no past admissions can be overlooked
Upper-extremity function assessment [87]	Objective Quick (physical task performed in less than 1 minute)	Does not assess cognitive impairment, depression, and comorbidity
Fried index [88]	Performance based Feasible in large populations	Floor effect (i.e., immobile patients)

The Fried index [88] identified frailty as 3 or more of the following: unintentional weight loss (10 pounds in preceding year), self-reported exhaustion, grip strength weakness, slow walking speed and decreased physical activity. The frailty phenotype per the Fried index is predictive of events in the following 3 years including incident falls, worsening mobility, hospitalizations, and deaths (hazard ratios range from 1.82 to 4.46). If less than 3 criteria are present, then the Fried index is predictive of frailty in 3–4 years of outpatient follow-up (OR 4.51).

A challenge of managing the frail elderly is the fact that frailty often leads to a complex presentation encompassing multiple diseases at once, e.g., delirium and immobility. The importance of identifying frailty is exemplified by the increased risk of adverse outcomes in this population as well as the need to focus on the patient and family goals as opposed to exposing frail patients to potential hazards. On the other hand, the degree to which frailty predicts procedural outcomes is called into question with the results of a study on outcomes after ileoanal pouch surgery in frail and older adults [89]. Frailty in this surgical study was based on the presence of chronic obstructive pulmonary disease, diabetes, hypertension, congestive heart failure, dependent functional status, and $\geq 10\%$ weight loss in preceding 6 months. Patients with no frailty traits versus >1 frailty traits revealed no greater difference in complications or mean hospital length of stay.

Gilbert et al. developed a frailty risk score from overrepresented ICD-10 diagnostic codes in a population of elderly patients with characteristics of frailty [86]. Their Hospital Frailty Risk Score was tested on two separate validation cohorts to assess prediction of adverse outcomes after emergency admission and identification of similarly frail individuals. The authors found that their hospital frailty risk score predicted increased 30 day mortality (OR 1.71 95% CI 1.68–1.75), longer hospital stay (OR 6.03 CI 5.92–6.10) and 30 day re-admission rate (OR 1.48 CI 1.46–1.50). An important limitation is that the use of ICD-10 codes does not fully capture disease severity and variation in documentation can contribute to measurement error.

Upper extremity range of motion and muscle fatigue are features of frailty. The upper-extremity function (UEF) test involves placement of wearable motion sensors to measure forearm and upper-arm motion to quantify slowness, weakness, exhaustion, flexibility, and frailty. A study by Toosizadeh et al. [87] involving 352 participants, validated the UEF test against the Fried frailty index. The UEF test accurately predicted Fried frailty criteria. Of note, the UEF test does not measure cognition. Similar to the Fried index, it lacks components of cognitive impairment, depression, and comorbidity.

Reducing CRC Risk While Medically Managing IBD in the Elderly Patient

There is conflicting evidence as to whether or not certain therapies for IBD can be chemoprotective. While aminosalicylates have been associated with a reduction in the development of all cancers including CRC, more recent studies show no reduction in risk of CRC [21, 90]. Nevertheless, most physicians will still recommend 5-ASA agents at a dose of at least 1.5 g/day. Side effects to look out for in the elderly include nephrotoxicity in the setting of baseline renal dysfunction, as well as concomitant use of 5-ASA with warfarin. Other medications used for IBD long-term and maintenance treatment are the thiopurines, azathioprine and 6-mercaptopurine. While there is thought that thiopurines increase the risk of malignancy by direct alterations in DNA, activation of oncogenes, and reduction in immune system surveillance of malignancy cells, studies have shown a reduced risk in CRN, especially in patients with a long disease duration greater than 8 years [91]. Reduced risk of CRN can be explained by a better control of inflammation. However, there is an increased risk of site-specific cancers with thiopurine use, specifically non-melanoma skin cancer and lymphoma.

In a retrospective cohort study of nearly 37,000 patients, the incidence rate of lymphoma was 2.31 per 1000 patients who were treated with thiopurines vs 0.6 per 1000 patients who had not been treated with thiopurines [92]. The incidence rate of lymphoma increases with duration of thiopurine therapy. The risk of lymphoproliferative disorders increases with age. In a systematic review of IBD patients using thiopurine therapy, patients had a moderately increased risk of non-melanoma skin cancer proportional to therapy duration [93]. With regards to age, there is a bimodal risk distribution where those between the ages of 30–50 and those over 70 had the greatest non-melanoma skin cancer risk. A multicenter retrospective cohort study of patients with IBD showed the frequency of extra-colonic cancer was higher in the elderly than in adults [94]. These factors are important to consider when balancing with the benefits of immunosuppressive treatment of IBD and potential reduction in CRN risk.

There is some evidence that ursodeoxycholic acid (UDCA) at a low dosage may reduce CRC risk by decreasing the exposure of colonic epithelial cells to carcinogenic bile acids. The American College of Gastroenterology suggests consideration of UDCA in daily divided doses of 13–15 mg/kg for colorectal neoplasia prevention, but studies have only focused on this benefit in IBD patients with PSC. Furthermore, small observational studies have shown that the benefit of UDCA in chemoprevention did not reach statistical significance when a 10–15 mg/kg dose was compared to placebo and a higher dose (28–30 mg/kg) significantly increased the risk of CRC in patients with PSC [30].

Patients taking sulfasalazine should be on folate supplementation as low folate intake has been associated with alteration of DNA and subsequent development of CRC [21]. As statins inhibit 3-hydroxy-3-methylglutaryl-coenzyme A (HMG-CoA) reductase, an enzyme overexpressed in cancer cells, there is thought that statins can help protect against CRC. In sporadic CRC, the chemoprotective effect has been modest (RR = 0.9) [30]. In the IBD patient, statin use is independently and inversely associated with CRC (odds ratio 0.42). However, statins are not incorporated into routine practice given the lack prospective studies.

Summary

Advanced age is a risk factor for CRC and development of adenomatous polyps. Recurrence after screening colonoscopy is unaffected by age. The risks of screening procedures may take precedence with greater comorbidities in the elderly population including functional status and consideration of patient preference. Additionally, there is greater risk of poor bowel prep given the known lower compliance rate in the elderly population. Nevertheless, consideration of individualized risk factors on a case-by-case basis will help decide which patients are candidates for screening in this challenging population.

Appendix

Table 11.4 Colorectal cancer screening options, pros and cons

Form of test	Mechanism	Pros	Cons	Sensitivity/specificity
Breath test				
Volatile organic compound analysis	Searches for unique cancer-related metabolomic patterns or volatile organic compound analysis in breath. Technique can also be used on urine, fecal, and blood samples	Low patient discomfort, high accuracy	High cost of gas chromatography and low manageability	85–86% sensitivity for CRC and 83–94% specificity for CRC [45, 50], 94% sensitivity and specificity for adenomas [48]

(continued)

Table 11.4 (continued)

Form of test	Mechanism	Pros	Cons	Sensitivity/specificity
Blood test				
Epi proColon	DNA mutations (mSEPT9, ß-actin) in a 10 ml blood sample	Patients may be more receptive to blood test	Less sensitive for CRC and advanced adenomas compared to FIT-DNA, not recommended by the Multi-Society Task Force	Pooled sensitivity and specificity for CRC is 71% and 92%, respectively. Sensitivity for adenomas ≥1 cm is 23%
Stool tests				
Guaiac-based fecal occult blood test (gFOBT)	Chemical guaiac to detect blood in stool	Inexpensive, safe, easy	Dietary peroxidases from foods may confound results, requires multiple samples; single digital FOBT is not recommended	Once-only test sensitivity for advanced neoplasia 24–50% at most, PPV of 3–10%
Fecal immunochemical test (FIT)	Antibodies to detect blood in stool	Fewer fecal samples required compared to FOBT	Low sensitivity for detecting polyps, must be done yearly	79–91% sensitivity, 88–94% specificity for CRC
FIT-DNA test (also referred to as the stool DNA test or Cologuard)	Combines FIT with a test that detects altered DNA in the stool	Higher sensitivity than FIT for CRC	Detects fewer than half of all large advanced adenomas limiting preventive role, lower specificity compared to FIT	92% sensitivity for CRC, 42% sensitivity for large advanced adenomas, specificity 87–90%
Endoscopy				
Flexible sigmoidoscopy (FS)	Identifies polyps or cancer in the rectum and lower third of the colon	Well tolerated without sedation, effective at reducing CRC mortality in distal colon cancer	Benefit limited to distal colon; if a precancerous polyp or cancer is found, colonoscopy is required for evaluation of the entire colon	Sensitivity of FS for detecting CRC in the entire colon was 58–75% [65]
Colonoscopy (optical colonoscopy)	Searches for polyps or cancer in the entire colon; provides opportunity for removal of most polyps and some cancers	Removal of polyps at time of exam is therapeutic, ability to visualize entire colon	Requires full bowel preparation and sedation (in the United States), expensive, patient requires escort upon going home	Sensitivity, specificity, and positive and negative predictive values for dysplasia optical diagnosis were 70%, 90%, 58%, and 94%, respectively [73] Rate of missed CRC 5.8% for non-IBD patients compared with 15.1% for CD and 15.8% for UC patients [4]

Table 11.4 (continued)

Form of test	Mechanism	Pros	Cons	Sensitivity/specificity
Colon capsule endoscopy	Minimally invasive tool that visualizes the colon via wireless camera in a capsule swallowed by the patient	Assesses mucosal inflammation	Cannot provide histologic evidence, risk of capsule retention in strictures, 9% technical failures [48]	Sensitivity of 71–73% for detection of all polyps and a specificity of 75–88% for polyps 6 mm or larger and specificity of 82–86% for more than 3 polyps
Radiology				
CT colonography (virtual colonoscopy)	Produces images of the entire colon using X-rays displayed on a computer screen for analysis	Less perforation risk compared to colonoscopy, can be done on anticoagulated patients, detection of extra-colonic findings (abdominal aortic aneurysm, renal cell carcinoma)	Lower sensitivity for polyps <8 mm compared to colonoscopy, requires bowel prep, procedure insufflation discomfort, contrast allergy, radiation exposure, need for colonoscopy if positive findings; should not be test of choice for IBD patients given no ability to detect flat lesions	66.8% sensitivity and 80.3% specificity for polyps, sensitivity for CRC 96%
MR colonography	Images the entire colon using magnetic fields	No radiation exposure, high soft-tissue contrast, noninvasive	Requires colonic distension, false positives from fecal residue, false negatives, misses flat lesions; limited data for use in IBD patients	Sensitivity and specificity of 88–90.9% and 96–98.5% for adenomas larger than 10 mm, sensitivity of 100% for detection of colorectal carcinoma [39]
Double-contrast barium enema	Barium and air are inserted through the rectum to visualize the rectum and colon	No longer in favor given patient discomfort as well as low sensitivity for polyp and CRC detection		Sensitivity 48% for CRC [33]

Table 11.5 Risk factors for colorectal cancer in patients with IBD

Risk factors	Comments
Younger age at onset	IBD patients develop CRC at younger age compared to patients with sporadic CRC (mean age 40–50 years vs 60 years) Diagnosis of UC < 19 years of age is associated with a RR of CRC of 43.8 compared to 2.65 in those 20–39. No studies have compared the RR of CRC in the elderly patient with IBD
Duration of disease	Duration of disease is only a proxy measure for cumulative inflammation burden which may not be accurate in this age
Anatomic extent of disease	Standard incidence ratio for CRC is 14.2 for left-sided colitis compared to 33.1 for pancolitis in patients diagnosed with UC between ages of 15 and 29 [30]
Severity of inflammation	Assess active inflammation, endoscopically and histologically [70]. Cumulative risk burden is based on multiple surveillance episodes [25] This is the only modifiable risk factor for the development of CRN
Colonic stricture	The prevalence of CRC is high in IBD patients with newly developed strictures but the prevalence of dysplasia is not increased Strictures within the past 5 years qualifies patients at high risk according to ECCO and merits yearly surveillance
Postinflammatory polyps	Unclear if CRN risk associated with pseudopolyps is due to previous inflammation or changes in mucosal surface leading to difficulty identifying neoplastic lesions. Pseudopolyps is associated with an increased risk of CRC in UC (OR 2.5%) after adjusting for surveillance colonoscopy and IBD therapy [30]
Family history of sporadic CRC	The absolute risk of CRC development is highest (29%) in IBD patients with a first-degree relative with CRC diagnosis <50 years of age [30]
Concurrent primary sclerosing cholangitis	In PSC and IBD patients, 85–90% have UC and remaining have CD [30]. Odds ratio of developing dysplasia or cancer in UC patients with PSC is 4.8
Previous history of cancer	Independent risk factor for development of any cancer
Prior colorectal dysplasia or CRC	Associated with a 4–25-fold increase in risk of developing pouch neoplasia

Comment: There is also a significant correlation between the number of risk factors present and the cumulative risk of developing high-grade dysplasia or CRC [78]. Cumulative incidence of HGD/CRC at 1 and 5 years after initial LGD is 0 and 1.8% for no risk factors, 9.6 and 17.7% for one risk factor, and 29 and 53.4% for two risk factors

References

1. Noone AM, Howlader N, Krapcho M, Miller D, Brest A, Yu M, Ruhl J, Tatalovich Z, Mariotto A, Lewis DR, Chen HS, Feuer EJ, Cronin KA, editors. SEER cancer statistics review, 1975–2015. National Cancer Institute; 2018. Available from: https://seer.cancer.gov/csr/1975_2015/
2. Society AC. Colorectal cancer screening guidelines: American Cancer Society, Inc.; 2018. Available from: https://www.cancer.org/health-care-professionals/american-cancer-society-prevention-early-detection-guidelines/colorectal-cancer-screening-guidelines.html
3. Siegel RL, Miller KD, Fedewa SA, Ahnen DJ, Meester RGS, Barzi A, et al. Colorectal cancer statistics, 2017. CA Cancer J Clin. 2017;67(3):177–93.

4. Gaidos JK, Bickston SJ. How to optimize colon cancer surveillance in inflammatory bowel disease patients. Inflamm Bowel Dis. 2016;22(5):1219–30.
5. Lee SY, Song WH, Oh SC, Min BW, Lee SI. Anatomical distribution and detection rate of colorectal neoplasms according to age in the colonoscopic screening of a Korean population. Ann Surg Treat Res. 2018;94(1):36–43.
6. Siegel R, Desantis C, Jemal A. Colorectal cancer statistics, 2014. CA Cancer J Clin. 2014;64(2):104–17.
7. Maratt JK, Dickens J, Schoenfeld PS, Elta GH, Jackson K, Rizk D, et al. Factors associated with surveillance adenoma and sessile serrated polyp detection rates. Dig Dis Sci. 2017;62(12):3579–85.
8. Corley DA, Jensen CD, Marks AR, Zhao WK, de Boer J, Levin TR, et al. Variation of adenoma prevalence by age, sex, race, and colon location in a large population: implications for screening and quality programs. Clin Gastroenterol Hepatol. 2013;11(2):172–80.
9. Mouchli MA, Ouk L, Scheitel MR, Chaudhry AP, Felmlee-Devine D, Grill DE, et al. Colonoscopy surveillance for high risk polyps does not always prevent colorectal cancer. World J Gastroenterol. 2018;24(8):905–16.
10. Kahi CJ, Myers LJ, Slaven JE, Haggstrom D, Pohl H, Robertson DJ, et al. Lower endoscopy reduces colorectal cancer incidence in older individuals. Gastroenterology. 2014;146(3):718–25.e3.
11. Esteva M, Ruiz A, Ramos M, Casamitjana M, Sanchez-Calavera MA, Gonzalez-Lujan L, et al. Age differences in presentation, diagnosis pathway and management of colorectal cancer. Cancer Epidemiol. 2014;38(4):346–53.
12. Iida Y, Kawai K, Tsuno NH, Ishihara S, Yamaguchi H, Sunami E, et al. Proximal shift of colorectal cancer along with aging. Clin Colorectal Cancer. 2014;13(4):213–8.
13. Bouvier AM, Launoy G, Bouvier V, Rollot F, Manfredi S, Faivre J, et al. Incidence and patterns of late recurrences in colon cancer patients. Int J Cancer. 2015;137(9):2133–8.
14. Bardhan K, Liu K. Epigenetics and colorectal cancer pathogenesis. Cancers. 2013;5(2):676–713.
15. Stegeman I, de Wijkerslooth TR, Stoop EM, van Leerdam ME, Dekker E, van Ballegooijen M, et al. Colorectal cancer risk factors in the detection of advanced adenoma and colorectal cancer. Cancer Epidemiol. 2013;37(3):278–83.
16. Gathirua-Mwangi WG, Monahan P, Song Y, Zollinger TW, Champion VL, Stump TE, et al. Changes in adult BMI and waist circumference are associated with increased risk of advanced colorectal neoplasia. Dig Dis Sci. 2017;62(11):3177–85.
17. Nimmons D, Limdi JK. Elderly patients and inflammatory bowel disease. World J Gastrointest Pharmacol Ther. 2016;7(1):51–65.
18. Gisbert JP, Chaparro M. Systematic review with meta-analysis: inflammatory bowel disease in the elderly. Aliment Pharmacol Ther. 2014;39(5):459–77.
19. Manosa M, Calafat M, de Francisco R, Garcia C, Casanova MJ, Huelin P, et al. Phenotype and natural history of elderly onset inflammatory bowel disease: a multicentre, case-control study. Aliment Pharmacol Ther. 2018;47(5):605–14.
20. Dulai PS, Sandborn WJ, Gupta S. Colorectal cancer and dysplasia in inflammatory bowel disease: a review of disease epidemiology, pathophysiology, and management. Cancer Prev Res (Philadelphia, PA). 2016;9(12):887–94.
21. Wilson JC, Furlano RI, Jick SS, Meier CR. A population-based study examining the risk of malignancy in patients diagnosed with inflammatory bowel disease. J Gastroenterol. 2016;51(11):1050–62.
22. Kim ER, Chang DK. Colorectal cancer in inflammatory bowel disease: the risk, pathogenesis, prevention and diagnosis. World J Gastroenterol. 2014;20(29):9872–81.
23. Herszenyi L, Barabas L, Miheller P, Tulassay Z. Colorectal cancer in patients with inflammatory bowel disease: the true impact of the risk. Dig Dis (Basel, Switzerland). 2015;33(1):52–7.
24. Bojesen RD, Riis LB, Hogdall E, Nielsen OH, Jess T. Inflammatory bowel disease and small bowel cancer risk, clinical characteristics, and histopathology: a population-based study. Clin Gastroenterol Hepatol. 2017;15(12):1900–7.e2.

25. Choi CR, Al Bakir I, Ding NJ, Lee GH, Askari A, Warusavitarne J, et al. Cumulative burden of inflammation predicts colorectal neoplasia risk in ulcerative colitis: a large single-centre study. Gut. 2017;68(3):[Epub].
26. Taleban S, Elquza E, Gower-Rousseau C, Peyrin-Biroulet L. Cancer and inflammatory bowel disease in the elderly. Dig Liver Dis. 2016;48(10):1105–11.
27. Ricciuto A, Kamath BM, Griffiths AM. The IBD and PSC phenotypes of PSC-IBD. Curr Gastroenterol Rep. 2018;20(4):16.
28. Folseraas T, Boberg KM. Cancer risk and surveillance in primary sclerosing cholangitis. Clin Liver Dis. 2016;20(1):79–98.
29. Liu G, Lin J, Xie H, Shen B, Stocchi L, Liu X. Histomorphological features and prognosis of colitis-associated colorectal cancer in patients with primary sclerosing cholangitis. Scand J Gastroenterol. 2015;50(11):1389–96.
30. Pulusu SSR, Lawrance IC. Dysplasia and colorectal cancer surveillance in inflammatory bowel disease. Expert Rev Gastroenterol Hepatol. 2017;11(8):711–22.
31. Sorensen JO, Nielsen OH, Andersson M, Ainsworth MA, Ytting H, Belard E, et al. Inflammatory bowel disease with primary sclerosing cholangitis: a Danish population-based cohort study 1977–2011. Liver Int. 2018;38(3):532–41.
32. Pickhardt PJ. Emerging stool-based and blood-based non-invasive DNA tests for colorectal cancer screening: the importance of cancer prevention in addition to cancer detection. Abdom Radiol (New York). 2016;41(8):1441–4.
33. Issa IA, Noureddine M. Colorectal cancer screening: an updated review of the available options. World J Gastroenterol. 2017;23(28):5086–96.
34. Kahi CJ, Pohl H, Myers LJ, Mobarek D, Robertson DJ, Imperiale TF. Colonoscopy and colorectal cancer mortality in the veterans affairs health care system: a case-control study. Ann Intern Med. 2018;168(7):481–8.
35. Doubeni CA, Corley DA, Quinn VP, Jensen CD, Zauber AG, Goodman M, et al. Effectiveness of screening colonoscopy in reducing the risk of death from right and left colon cancer: a large community-based study. Gut. 2018;67(2):291–8.
36. Doroudi M, Schoen RE, Pinsky PF. Early detection versus primary prevention in the PLCO flexible sigmoidoscopy screening trial: which has the greatest impact on mortality? Cancer. 2017;123(24):4815–22.
37. Bevan RR, Rutter MD. Colorectal cancer screening – who, how, and when? Clin Endosc. 2018;51(1):37–49.
38. Duarte RB, Bernardo WM, Sakai CM, Silva GL, Guedes HG, Kuga R, et al. Computed tomography colonography versus colonoscopy for the diagnosis of colorectal cancer: a systematic review and meta-analysis. Ther Clin Risk Manag. 2018;14:349–60.
39. van der Paardt MP, Stoker J. Magnetic resonance colonography for screening and diagnosis of colorectal cancer. Magn Reson Imaging Clin N Am. 2014;22(1):67–83.
40. Graser A, Melzer A, Lindner E, Nagel D, Herrmann K, Stieber P, et al. Magnetic resonance colonography for the detection of colorectal neoplasia in asymptomatic adults. Gastroenterology. 2013;144(4):743–50.e2.
41. Levine MS, Yee J. History, evolution, and current status of radiologic imaging tests for colorectal cancer screening. Radiology. 2014;273(2 Suppl):S160–80.
42. Young GP, Symonds EL, Allison JE, Cole SR, Fraser CG, Halloran SP, et al. Advances in fecal occult blood tests: the FIT revolution. Dig Dis Sci. 2015;60(3):609–22.
43. Shaukat A, Mongin SJ, Geisser MS, Lederle FA, Bond JH, Mandel JS, et al. Long-term mortality after screening for colorectal cancer. N Engl J Med. 2013;369(12):1106–14.
44. Lauby-Secretan B, Vilahur N, Bianchini F, Guha N, Straif K. The IARC perspective on colorectal cancer screening. N Engl J Med. 2018;378(18):1734–40.
45. Di Lena M, Porcelli F, Altomare DF. Volatile organic compounds as new biomarkers for colorectal cancer: a review. Colorectal Dis. 2016;18(7):654–63.
46. Cha JM, Suh M, Kwak MS, Sung NY, Choi KS, Park B, et al. Risk of interval cancer in fecal immunochemical test screening significantly higher during the summer months: results from

the National Cancer Screening Program in Korea. Am J Gastroenterol. 2018;113(4):611–21.
47. Imperiale TF, Ransohoff DF, Itzkowitz SH, Levin TR, Lavin P, Lidgard GP, Ahlquist DA, Berger BM. Multitarget stool DNA testing for colorectal-cancer screening. N Engl J Med. 2014;370:1287–97.
48. Rex D. Colorectal cancer screening: recommendations for physicians and patients from the U.S. Multi-Society Task Force on Colorectal Cancer. Gastroenterology. 2017;153(1):307–23.
49. Sole X, Crous-Bou M, Cordero D, Olivares D, Guino E, Sanz-Pamplona R, et al. Discovery and validation of new potential biomarkers for early detection of colon cancer. PLoS One. 2014;9(9):e106748.
50. Amal H, Leja M, Funka K, Lasina I, Skapars R, Sivins A, et al. Breath testing as potential colorectal cancer screening tool. Int J Cancer. 2016;138(1):229–36.
51. Lopez A, Collet-Fenetrier B, Belle A, Peyrin-Biroulet L. Patients' knowledge and fear of colorectal cancer risk in inflammatory bowel disease. J Dig Dis. 2016;17(6):383–91.
52. Kumar A. Effect of functional status on the quality of bowel preparation in elderly patients undergoing screening and surveillance colonoscopy. Gut Liver. 2016;10(4):569–73.
53. Senore C, Correale L, Regge D, Hassan C, Iussich G, Silvani M, et al. Flexible sigmoidoscopy and CT colonography screening: patients' experience with and factors for undergoing screening-insight from the proteus colon trial. Radiology. 2018;286(3):873–83.
54. Childers RE, Williams JL, Sonnenberg A. Practice patterns of sedation for colonoscopy. Gastrointest Endosc. 2015;82(3):503–11.
55. Lin OS. Performing colonoscopy in elderly and very elderly patients: risks, costs and benefits. World J Gastrointest Endosc. 2014;6(6):220–6.
56. Kanonidou Z, Karystianou G. Anesthesia for the elderly. Hippokratia. 2007;11(4):175–7.
57. Al-Zubaidi AM, Al-Shadadi AA, Alghamdy HU, Alzobady AH, Al-Qureshi LA, Al-Bakri IM. Retrospective comparison of sedated and non-sedated colonoscopy in an outpatient practice. Indian J Gastroenterol. 2016;35(2):129–32.
58. Ogawa T, Ohda Y, Nagase K, Kono T, Tozawa K, Tomita T, et al. Evaluation of discomfort during colonoscopy with conventional and ultrathin colonoscopes in ulcerative colitis patients. Dig Endosc. 2015;27(1):99–105.
59. Sofi AA, Nawras A, Khan MA, Howden CW, Lee WM. Meta-analysis of the performance of ultrathin vs. standard colonoscopes. Endoscopy. 2017;49(4):351–8.
60. Dorreen A, Heisler C, Jones J. Treatment of inflammatory bowel disease in the older patient. Inflamm Bowel Dis. 2018;24(6):1155–66.
61. Razavi F, Gross S, Katz S. Endoscopy in the elderly: risks, benefits, and yield of common endoscopic procedures. Clin Geriatr Med. 2014;30(1):133–47.
62. Johnson DA, Lieberman D, Inadomi JM, Ladabaum U, Becker RC, Gross SA, et al. Increased post-procedural non-gastrointestinal adverse events after outpatient colonoscopy in high-risk patients. Clin Gastroenterol Hepatol. 2017;15(6):883–91.e9.
63. Garcia-Albeniz X, Hsu J, Bretthauer M, Hernan MA. Effectiveness of screening colonoscopy to prevent colorectal cancer among Medicare beneficiaries aged 70 to 79 years a prospective observational study. Ann Intern Med. 2017;166(1):18–26.
64. Rathore F, Sultan N, Byrne D. Tolerance of colonoscopy and questioning its utility in the elderly population. Ir Med J. 2014;107(8):247.
65. Zhang J, Cheng Z, Ma Y, He C, Lu Y, Zhao Y, et al. Effectiveness of screening modalities in colorectal cancer: a network meta-analysis. Clin Colorectal Cancer. 2017;16(4):252–63.
66. Yoshida N, Naito Y, Murakami T, Hirose R, Ogiso K, Inada Y, et al. Safety and efficacy of a same-day low-volume 1 L PEG bowel preparation in colonoscopy for the elderly people and people with renal dysfunction. Dig Dis Sci. 2016;61(11):3229–35.
67. Saltzman JR, Cash BD, Pasha SF, Early DS, Muthusamy VR, Khashab MA, et al. Bowel preparation before colonoscopy. Gastrointest Endosc. 2015;81(4):781–94.
68. Moreno C, Kim DH, Bartel TB, Cash BD, Chang KJ, Feig BW, et al. ACR appropriateness criteria((R)) colorectal cancer screening. J Am Coll Radiol. 2018;15(5s):S56–s68.
69. Matsuoka K, Kobayashi T, Ueno F, Matsui T, Hirai F, Inoue N, et al. Evidence-based clinical

practice guidelines for inflammatory bowel disease. J Gastroenterol. 2018;53(3):305–53.

70. Yu JX, East JE, Kaltenbach T. Surveillance of patients with inflammatory bowel disease. Best Pract Res Clin Gastroenterol. 2016;30(6):949–58.

71. Huguet JM, Suárez P, Ferrer-Barceló L, et al. Endoscopic recommendations for colorectal cancer screening and surveillance in patients with inflammatory bowel disease: review of general recommendations. World J Gastrointest Endosc. 2017;9(6):255–62.

72. Ten Hove JR, Mooiweer E, Dekker E, van der Meulen-de Jong AE, Offerhaus GJ, Ponsioen CY, et al. Low rate of dysplasia detection in mucosa surrounding dysplastic lesions in patients undergoing surveillance for inflammatory bowel diseases. Clin Gastroenterol Hepatol. 2017;15(2):222–8.e2.

73. Carballal S, Maisterra S, Lopez-Serrano A, Gimeno-Garcia AZ, Vera MI, Marin-Garbriel JC, et al. Real-life chromoendoscopy for neoplasia detection and characterisation in long-standing IBD. Gut. 2018;67(1):70–8.

74. Lichtenstein GR, Loftus EV, Isaacs KL, Regueiro MD, Gerson LB, Sands BE. ACG clinical guideline: management of Crohn's disease in adults. Am J Gastroenterol. 2018;113(4):481–517.

75. Cohen-Mekelburg S, Schneider Y, Gold S, Scherl E, Steinlauf A. Advances in the diagnosis and management of colonic dysplasia in patients with inflammatory bowel disease. Gastroenterol Hepatol. 2017;13(6):357–62.

76. Lin JS, Piper MA, Perdue LA, Rutter C, Webber EM, O'Connor E, et al. U.S. Preventive Services Task Force Evidence Syntheses, formerly Systematic Evidence Reviews. Screening for colorectal cancer: a systematic review for the US Preventive Services Task Force. Rockville: Agency for Healthcare Research and Quality (US); 2016.

77. Cha JM. Would you recommend screening colonoscopy for the very elderly? Intest Res. 2014;12(4):275–80.

78. Bye WA, Nguyen TM, Parker CE, Jairath V, East JE. Strategies for detecting colon cancer in patients with inflammatory bowel disease. Cochrane Database Syst Rev. 2017;9:CD000279.

79. Eluri S, Parian AM, Limketkai BN, Ha CY, Brant SR, Dudley-Brown S, et al. Nearly a third of high-grade dysplasia and colorectal cancer is undetected in patients with inflammatory bowel disease. Dig Dis Sci. 2017;62(12):3586–93.

80. van Hees F, Saini SD, Lansdorp-Vogelaar I, Vijan S, Meester RG, de Koning HJ, et al. Personalizing colonoscopy screening for elderly individuals based on screening history, cancer risk, and comorbidity status could increase cost effectiveness. Gastroenterology. 2015;149(6):1425–37.

81. Yourman LC, Lee SJ, Schonberg MA, Widera EW, Smith AK. Prognostic indices for older adults: a systematic review. JAMA. 2012;307(2):182–92.

82. Weigl K, et al. Strongly enhanced colorectal cancer risk stratification enhanced by combining family history and genetic risk scores. Clin Epidemiol. 2018;10:143–52.

83. Imperiale TF, Yu M, Monahan PO, Stump TE, Tabbey R, Glowinski E, et al. Risk of advanced neoplasia using the National Cancer Institute's colorectal cancer risk assessment tool. J Natl Cancer Inst. 2017;109(1):1.

84. Cha JM, Kozarek RA, La Selva D, Gluck M, Ross A, Chiorean M, et al. Risks and benefits of colonoscopy in patients 90 years or older, compared with younger patients. Clin Gastroenterol Hepatol. 2016;14(1):80–6.e1.

85. Maratt JK, Lewis CL, Saffar D, Weston LE, Myers A, Piper MS, et al. Veterans' attitudes towards deintensification of surveillance colonoscopy for low-risk adenomas. Clin Gastroenterol Hepatol. 2018;16(12):1999–2000.

86. Gilbert T, Neuburger J, Kraindler J, Keeble E, Smith P, Ariti C, et al. Development and validation of a Hospital Frailty Risk Score focusing on older people in acute care settings using electronic hospital records: an observational study. Lancet (London, England). 2018;391(10132):1775–82.

87. Toosizadeh N, Wendel C, Hsu C-H, Zamrini E, Mohler J. Frailty assessment in older adults using upper-extremity function: index development. BMC Geriatr. 2017;17(1):117.

88. Fried LP, Tangen CM, Walston J, Newman AB, Hirsch C, Gottdiener J, et al. Frailty in older

adults: evidence for a phenotype. J Gerontol A Biol Sci Med Sci. 2001;56(3):M146–56.
89. Cohan JN, Bacchetti P, Varma MG, Finlayson E. Outcomes after ileoanal pouch surgery in frail and older adults. J Surg Res. 2015;198(2):327–33.
90. Qiu X, Ma J, Wang K, Zhang H. Chemopreventive effects of 5-aminosalicylic acid on inflammatory bowel disease-associated colorectal cancer and dysplasia: a systematic review with meta-analysis. Oncotarget. 2017;8(1):1031–45.
91. Zhu Z, Mei Z, Guo Y, Wang G, Wu T, Cui X, et al. Reduced risk of inflammatory bowel disease-associated colorectal neoplasia with use of thiopurines: a systematic review and meta-analysis. J Crohns Colitis. 2018;12(5):546–58.
92. Khan N, Abbas AM, Lichtenstein GR, Loftus EV Jr, Bazzano LA. Risk of lymphoma in patients with ulcerative colitis treated with thiopurines: a nationwide retrospective cohort study. Gastroenterology. 2013;145(5):1007–15.e3.
93. Hagen JW, Pugliano-Mauro MA. Nonmelanoma skin cancer risk in patients with inflammatory bowel disease undergoing thiopurine therapy: a systematic review of the literature. Dermatol Sur. 2018;44(4):469–80.
94. Hou JK, Feagins LA, Waljee AK. Characteristics and behavior of elderly-onset inflammatory bowel disease: a multi-center US study. Inflamm Bowel Dis. 2016;22(9):2200–5.

Chapter 12
Use of Biologic Drugs Following an Initial Diagnosis of Malignancy

Jordan Axelrad, Shannon Chang, and David Hudesman

As the population of patients with inflammatory bowel disease (IBD) increases and ages, there is an inevitable increase in the risk of cancer development [1]. Gastroenterologists and oncologists caring for patients with IBD and cancer are increasingly confronted with questions regarding the management of IBD after a diagnosis of cancer [2].

Given the evidence-based and theoretical risks of therapy-associated malignancy, patients with a history of cancer were excluded from clinical trials of IBD medications. Additionally, there is substantial data within the solid organ transplant literature indicating that immunosuppression, specifically thiopurine and calcineurin inhibitors, increases the risk of new and recurrent malignancies in patients with a history of cancer [3, 4]. This risk seems directly correlated with time from cancer diagnosis where transplantation less than 5 years from a cancer diagnosis is associated with a nearly threefold greater risk of cancer recurrence compared to transplantation more than 5 years from a cancer diagnosis [5].

As such, oncologists and gastroenterologists generally suspend immunosuppression for IBD after a diagnosis of cancer; however, this approach may worsen IBD and even complicate cancer management. Several studies have demonstrated a major modification in IBD medications after a diagnosis of cancer [2, 6, 7]. In a French observational study, a diagnosis of extra-intestinal cancer had a marked impact on the management of IBD, with a lesser use of thiopurines (19% vs 25%, $p < 0.001$) and an increased use of intestinal surgery (4.0% vs 2.5%, $p = 0.05$), but was not associated with significant modifications in activity of IBD [6].

J. Axelrad · S. Chang
NYU School of Medicine, New York, NY, USA
e-mail: Jordan.axelrad@nyulangone.org; Shannon.chang@nyulangone.org

D. Hudesman (✉)
NYU School of Medicine, New York, NY, USA

Inflammatory Bowel Disease Center, NYU Langone Health, New York, NY, USA
e-mail: david.hudesman@nyulangone.org

© Springer Nature Switzerland AG 2019   165
J. D. Feuerstein, A. S. Cheifetz (eds.), *Cancer Screening in Inflammatory Bowel Disease*, https://doi.org/10.1007/978-3-030-15301-4_12

Although there is very limited population-based data on the use of immunosuppression in patients with IBD and a history of cancer, emerging data may suggest safety. In a French prospective observational cohort, exposure to immunosuppression was independently associated with the development of cancer with an adjusted hazard ratio (HR) of 1.9 (95% CI: 1.2–3.0); however, it did not increase the risk of new or recurrent cancer in patients with a history of cancer [8]. Given the limited number of patients with IBD and a history of cancer with subsequent exposure to immunosuppression in the cohort, this conclusion only applied to thiopurine exposure and no conclusions were drawn on anti-TNF-α therapies [8].

In a similar observational study in the United States, nearly 30% of patients with IBD and a history of cancer developed new or recurrent cancer, however, exposure to TNF-α antagonists, thiopurines, or the combination was not associated with an increased risk of new or recurrent cancer within 5 years following a diagnosis of cancer (Log-rank $p = 0.14$) [9]. In addition, duration of TNF-α antagonists after a diagnosis of cancer was not associated with the risk or type of new or recurrent cancer [9]. In a small study of 79 refractory IBD patients with previous malignancy diagnosed within 17 months, exposure to anti-TNF therapy yielded only a mild risk of incident cancer (crude incidence rate 84.5, 95% CI: 83.1–85.8 per 1000 patient-years) [10].

In a meta-analysis of 16 studies comprising 11,702 persons with an immune-mediated disease contributing 31,258 person-years of follow-up evaluation after a diagnosis of cancer, there were similar rates of cancer recurrence among individuals with prior cancer who received no immunosuppression, anti-TNF therapy, immune-modulator therapy, or combination treatments [11].

There are few data regarding the concomitant use of IBD therapies during active malignancy, most limited to small case series or case reports. There is emerging data regarding the intermittent use of TNF antagonists and anti-integrins for colitis mediated by immune checkpoint inhibitors, cancer therapy now commonly used for a variety of malignancy types [2, 12–14]. These limited data suggest biologics may be safely used during active malignancy and active chemotherapy; however, robust prospective data in patients with IBD on long-term immunosuppression are lacking.

In practice, the decision to use biologic therapy in a patient with a history of cancer is made on a case-by-case basis. Given existing safety data, we recommend considering anti-integrin or anti-IL12/23 agents in patients with a history of cancer who require biologic agents. However, in patients who fail these agents or in patients who are not expected to respond, anti-TNF therapies may be used in close consultation with an oncologist. In addition, surgery may be considered earlier in IBD management as appropriate.

References

1. Khan N, Vallarino C, Lissoos T, et al. Risk of malignancy in a nationwide cohort of elderly inflammatory bowel disease patients. Drugs Aging. 2017;34:859–68.
2. Axelrad JE, Lichtiger S, Yajnik V. Inflammatory bowel disease and cancer: the role of inflammation, immunosuppression, and cancer treatment. World J Gastroenterol. 2016;22:4794–801.
3. Penn I. Kidney transplantation in patients previously treated for renal carcinomas. Transpl Int. 1993;6:350.
4. Gutierrez-Dalmau A, Campistol JM. Immunosuppressive therapy and malignancy in organ transplant recipients: a systematic review. Drugs. 2007;67:1167–98.
5. Acuna SA, Huang JW, Dossa F, et al. Cancer recurrence after solid organ transplantation: a systematic review and meta-analysis. Transplant Rev. 2017;31:240–8.
6. Rajca S, Seksik P, Bourrier A, et al. Impact of the diagnosis and treatment of cancer on the course of inflammatory bowel disease. J Crohns Colitis. 2014;8:819–24.
7. Axelrad JE, Fowler SA, Friedman S, et al. Effects of cancer treatment on inflammatory bowel disease remission and reactivation. Clin Gastroenterol Hepatol. 2012;10:1021–7.e1.
8. Beaugerie L, Carrat F, Colombel J-F, et al. Risk of new or recurrent cancer under immunosuppressive therapy in patients with IBD and previous cancer. Gut. 2014;63:1416–23.
9. Axelrad J, Bernheim O, Colombel J-F, et al. Risk of new or recurrent cancer in patients with inflammatory bowel disease and previous cancer exposed to immunosuppressive and anti-tumor necrosis factor agents. Clin Gastroenterol Hepatol. 2016;14:58–64.
10. Poullenot F, Seksik P, Beaugerie L, et al. Risk of incident cancer in inflammatory bowel disease patients starting anti-TNF therapy while having recent malignancy. Inflamm Bowel Dis. 2016;22:1362–9.
11. Shelton E, Laharie D, Scott FI, et al. Cancer recurrence following immune-suppressive therapies in patients with immune-mediated diseases: a systematic review and meta-analysis. Gastroenterology. 2016;151:97–109.e4.
12. Bergqvist V, Hertervig E, Gedeon P, et al. Vedolizumab treatment for immune checkpoint inhibitor-induced enterocolitis. Cancer Immunol Immunother. 2017;66:581–92.
13. Wang Y, Abu-Sbeih H, Mao E, et al. Immune-checkpoint inhibitor-induced diarrhea and colitis in patients with advanced malignancies: retrospective review at MD Anderson. J Immunother Cancer. 2018;6:37.
14. Geukes Foppen MH, Rozeman EA, van WS, et al. Immune checkpoint inhibition-related colitis: symptoms, endoscopic features, histology and response to management. ESMO Open. 2018;3:e000278.

Index

© Springer Nature Switzerland AG 2019   169
J. D. Feuerstein, A. S. Cheifetz (eds.), *Cancer Screening in Inflammatory Bowel
Disease*, https://doi.org/10.1007/978-3-030-15301-4

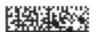